IMPORTANT NOTICE

This book is intended not as a substitute for personal medical advice but as a supplement to that advice for the patient who wishes to understand more about his or her condition.

Before taking any form of treatment YOU SHOULD ALWAYS CONSULT YOUR MEDICAL PRACTITIONER.

In particular (without limit) you should note that advances in medical science occur rapidly and some of the information about drugs and treatment contained in this booklet may very soon be out of date.

The author is most grateful to Alan Robertson, Consultant Obstetrician and Gynaecologist, and Nick Matthews, exercise scientist and physiotherapist, for their contributions on exercise in pregnancy and general physical conditioning.

Family Doctor Publications, PO Box 4664, Poole, Dorset BH15 1NN

Medical Editor: Dr Tony Smith
Consultant Editors: Chris McLaughlin, Lynne Low
Cover Artist: Dave Eastbury
Medical Artist: Angela Christie
Design: MPG Design, Blandford Forum, Dorset
Printing: Reflex Litho, Thetford, using acid-free paper

ISBN: 1 898205 57 4

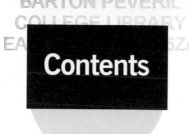

Contents

Introduction

Although the proliferation of magazines, newspaper articles and TV programmes devoted to fitness might suggest that more and more people are taking up exercise, the reality is very different. Many people get hardly any exercise at all, travelling everywhere by car or public transport and never using the stairs when a lift or escalator is available. In fact, many more people watch sport than actually take part in it.

Health experts and Government advisory committees are constantly urging all of us to take more exercise, but is there really good evidence that doing so will benefit our health? The answer is a very definite yes. A mass of research studies has shown that men and women whose lives include some regular physical exertion feel better and are less prone to develop a whole range of conditions, from heart disease to osteoporosis (brittle bones). Forty years ago, a study in London showed that bus conductors who ran up and down stairs all day long had fewer heart attacks than their colleagues who sat down and drove the buses. Since then, many other researchers have confirmed that regular exercise reduces the chances of dying of heart disease. Not only are they healthier, but most people who exercise regularly also look leaner and in better shape.

In contrast, being physically inactive means that you find any kind of exertion a pain and you tire easily, regardless of your age. What is more, your muscles gradually become weaker and your bones less dense. If you do try to start jogging or playing tennis, for example, you become exhausted within a few minutes.

The longer you remain inactive,

the worse this state of unfitness becomes. Regular exercise, however, can turn it around at any age.

This book is in two sections. The first section sets out to explain what happens to the body during exercise, how its various systems respond to training, and why such changes are beneficial. The chapter on training explains what it is, and how to go about choosing the right programme for your needs. Exercise is only one part of healthy living, and the other components –

THE BENEFITS OF EXERCISE

- Your heart becomes stronger and works more efficiently
- You can lose weight if you combine exercise and healthy eating
- You feel better about yourself
- You are less likely to be anxious or depressed and feel more positive
- You may be able to bring down a slightly raised blood pressure to normal
- Your levels of cholesterol and other blood fats will be healthier
- You are likely to drink less alcohol and cut down or stop smoking
- Women are likely to have healthier pregnancies
- You are less likely to suffer from low back pain
- You will feel positive benefits if you have a specific health problem, such as lung disease, diabetes, arthritis or renal disease, or have had an organ transplantation
- You will find that it helps with your rehabilitation if you have cancer or are suffering the effects of cancer treatments
- You are less likely to be off work and achieve more while you're there

nutrition, rest, special dietary supplements and drug/alcohol use – are also discussed.

The second section deals with common sports and exercise-related problems and injuries, and how to avoid becoming a casualty. Specific injuries common to many sports are detailed, together with the appropriate treatment.

Everyone should exercise and, although the first-time aerobics class member and the marathon runner are at opposite ends of the spectrum, their problems and concerns are likely to be similar in some respects. We hope that you'll find this a useful guide whether you're an uncertain amateur, a regular weekend participant or someone for whom sport is far more than just a healthy pastime.

KEY POINTS

✓ Many people get hardly any exercise at all

✓ Men and women whose lives include some regular physical exertion feel better and are less susceptible to a wide range of illnesses

The body and exercise

Regular exercise leads to the heart becoming more efficient. The volume of blood pumped with each heart beat is increased, so the heart rate becomes slower, and therefore is more capable of speeding up during exertion. This is called the training effect. Top athletes have been known to have resting heart rates lower than 40 beats per minute (the average for an untrained person is about 72 beats per minute).

The training effect is one aspect of overall fitness, which enables the cardiovascular system and the lungs to supply blood and oxygen to the muscles more effectively and efficiently. These changes in fitness can be measured scientifically. The muscles show increased stamina, become stronger and contract more firmly, thus increasing their capacity for work and activity. Tendons surrounding joints become stronger, so that the joints are more stable and are thus less liable to injury – this is especially important in older people. The joints themselves become capable of an improved range of movement and are more flexible. Finally, the effects of age and chronic diseases including coronary artery disease are reduced.

WHAT IS FITNESS?

Total fitness is defined in the *Oxford Dictionary of Sports Science and Medicine* as: 'The ability of an individual to live a happy and well balanced life. It involves not only physical but also intellectual, emotional, social and spiritual aspects.'

Physical fitness by itself has several components. These are strength, speed, flexibility and endurance. Skill is also important in sports and exercise. It is something you learn, usually by repeating a range of pre-set movements. The skill factor is important in avoiding injury.

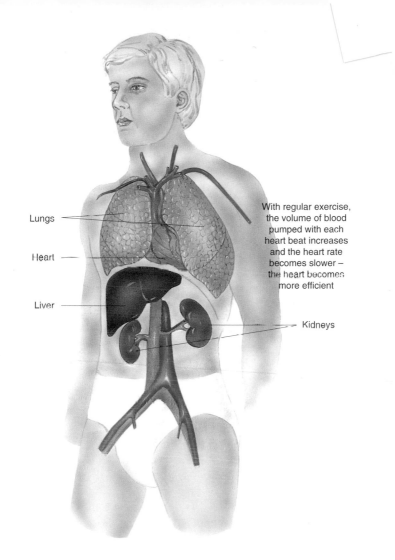

Lungs

Heart

Liver

With regular exercise, the volume of blood pumped with each heart beat increases and the heart rate becomes slower – the heart becomes more efficient

Kidneys

The training effect enables the cardiovascular system and the lungs to supply nutrients and oxygen to the muscles and vital organs more efficiently.

Strength

This is defined as the maximum force that a muscle or group of muscles can exert in a single contraction. In practical terms, the person who can lift 200 pounds (90 kilograms) has twice the strength of someone who can lift 100 pounds

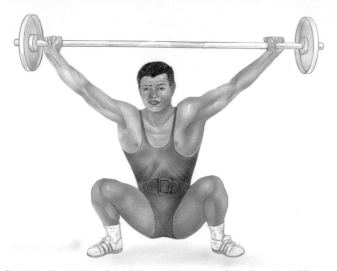

Strength – the maximum force that a muscle or group of muscles can exert in a single contraction.

(45 kg). Tests for muscle strength can be performed using special equipment such as strength-dynamometers, free weights or isokinetic strength-testing machinery. Weight-lifting and shot-putting are good examples of how strength is tested on the sports field. In other sports, certain movements are repeated over and over again; this also requires strength in the right places, for example, in the arms of tennis players.

Speed

This is defined and measured as the time taken to move a single limb (limb speed) or the total body (body speed) between two fixed points. It can be recorded simply as a time (in seconds) or, if the distance is known, it can be given units of velocity, that is, feet per second, metres per second, or whatever.

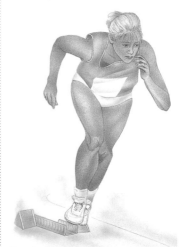

Speed – the time taken to move the body or a limb between two fixed points.

The time taken for a short sprint (less than 60 metres) or a karate chop is an example of a speed test. These can be measured by equipment such as lasers and light sensors.

Muscular power

Muscular power is strength and speed of movement combined. Mathematically, power equals strength times speed or force times velocity. For example, two people may be able to lift a 150-pound (68-kg) weight, but the one who can do it in half the time of the other has twice the power of the slower person. Power is a key component for most athletic performances. It determines, for example, how effectively a tennis player can serve, how far a golfer can drive a golf ball or whether a penalty kick beats the goalkeeper.

Flexibility

This is an aspect of fitness that is sometimes mistakenly overlooked. It is crucial in preventing injury – especially to muscles and ligaments – and should be an essential part of the training programme of all top-class performers. Training experts, both in the USA and in the UK, believe that a degree of overall body flexibility is desirable for everyone. Some of the more appealing aspects of flexibility are:

- It can be improved by practice

- It does not use up much energy

- It is safe and does not require apparatus

- It is enjoyable.

At least 15 to 20 minutes of flexibility and stretching exercises two to three times per week would be a valuable part of your overall fitness programme. There are two types of flexibility exercises: ballistic and static. Static flexibility exercises are preferable because they are much less likely to lead to injury.

Ballistic exercises involve activities such as bobbing or bouncing up and down, stretching

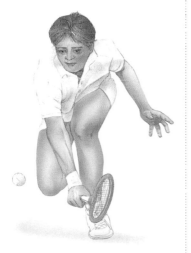

Power – the combination of speed of movement and strength.

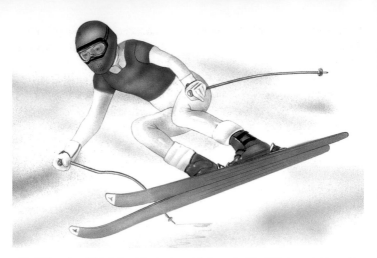

Flexibility – the ability to bend the body and limbs easily. Flexibility is crucial to avoid injury, especially to muscles and ligaments.

the inner aspects of the thighs and rapid rotational exercises of the trunk for the abdominal and back muscles. Although they are effective, you have less control over them than in static stretching and they can cause a muscle reflex which may limit your movements.

Static exercises are controlled stretching movements. To achieve the desired effect, you need to do them for only 20 to 30 minutes two or three times a week. They require little energy and are safe. You simply move your body slowly to the stretched position until you feel a slight discomfort, then hold the stretch position for up to 20 seconds. Remember to stay relaxed, keep breathing and focus your attention on the part that you are stretching (see pages 30–3).

WHAT HAPPENS TO THE BODY DURING EXERCISE?

Muscles need energy to contract, and this comes from food that is broken down to form energy stores in the muscles, liver and fat. The body produces energy from these stores in two different ways:

- by aerobic means (requiring oxygen)

- by anaerobic means (not requiring oxygen).

The process involved is called metabolism.

Anaerobic energy is used for short bursts of activity such as sprinting, lifting or jumping. Once anaerobic energy is used up, it cannot be replenished quickly.

There are two anaerobic pathways: for the first few seconds of high intensity activity (for example, a 100-metre sprint), what is called the phosphogen system is used. Beyond these first few seconds, two other systems take over to release energy for further muscular contractions and relaxations. These are known as anaerobic glycolysis and the oxidative system (aerobic energy production). Anaerobic glycolysis will supply energy in all-out sprint events for one or two minutes, but it leads to an accumulation of lactic acid in the muscle and body fluids, halting the process of glycogen breakdown that is responsible for supplying anaerobic energy. After that, aerobic energy is required because without this our ability to exercise would be limited to only a few minutes.

Aerobic energy is used for longer sessions of exertion, such as medium- and long-distance running, swimming and brisk walking. This energy can be continuously produced to meet the body's needs during exercise, but not at the high rate supplied by anaerobic metabolism. The term 'anaerobic threshold' is used to define the point at which the body cannot meet the energy demands placed upon it by the aerobic pathways. The body then starts to work anaerobically and produces lactic acid and other metabolic poisons.

It is the way the body produces and uses both these kinds of energy that is changed by increasing fitness. When you are fit, all the systems in your body are adapted towards producing and using energy in the most efficient way possible.

During prolonged exercise, anaerobic energy is used first. However, your body starts to adapt to the exertion by trying to maintain a good supply of oxygen to the muscles to allow aerobic metabolism to take place. For this, your heart has to beat faster and your lungs have to take in faster and deeper breaths so that the red blood cells carrying oxygen to your muscles are pumped faster towards their destination.

Various other changes also occur to ensure that your muscles get the blood supply they need – for instance, blood flow to your intestines and kidneys is decreased so that your muscles get a bigger share of the blood supply. Fitness and training reduce the need for such changes (which are stressful for the body) to take place early, so they will be needed only after you've been exercising for a long time. Instead, your heart, lungs, muscles and blood supply are all adapted to 'make light' of the exercise – they have a reserve capacity for exertion, and you don't

Surplus energy is stored as fat in adipose tissue

A small quantity of energy, for immediate and high-intensity activity, is stored within the muscles themselves

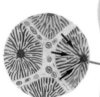

Heart

Liver

Stomach

Surplus energy from digested food is stored in the liver as glycogen

Food is digested in the stomach and intestine and the nutrients absorbed

Muscles need energy to contract, and this comes from food that is broken down and stored in the muscles, liver and fat.

start to experience discomfort and fatigue until much later.

If you rarely exert yourself beyond a certain point, you may kid yourself that you are fit because you only ever do things in short bursts, and so always use anaerobic energy. If, however, you were to run for longer, your heart rate would increase uncomfortably, you would quickly become out of breath, your muscles would weaken and tire, and you would soon have to stop. Someone who is fit, however, would be adapted to keep producing aerobic energy for their muscles, and their heart and lungs would work more efficiently to keep supplying the oxygen required for this.

Although it supplies energy more slowly, unit for unit, aerobic energy production releases almost ten times more energy than anaerobic means. Aerobic energy is also 'cleaner' – it produces mainly water and carbon dioxide as by-products. Aerobic metabolism produces less lactic acid – it is thought that the accumulation of lactic acid in the muscle is one reason for muscle fatigue and pain, the rising acidity progressively inhibiting further metabolism.

Energy sources

For competitive athletes, a correct fitness training programme is crucial because they have different patterns of energy requirements and need particular combinations of muscle use, depending on their particular sport. If, however, you just want to maintain your level of fitness, you can adopt a more relaxed programme which combines aerobic and anaerobic fitness, some strength and flexibility training, and relaxation (see later under 'All about training').

WHAT IS FATIGUE?

As mentioned above, muscle fatigue is thought to result partly from the accumulation of lactic acid from anaerobic metabolism. Other

ENERGY SOURCES	
Energy source	**Duration of energy source**
Anaerobic	
Intramuscular phosphogen	Few seconds
Intramuscular glycogen	Up to 50 seconds
Aerobic	
Glycogen	2 hours (continuous moderate-to-high intensity exercise)
Fat	Days
Protein	Protein can be an energy source at extremes of exertion and endurance

causes are the depletion of energy stores in the muscle (for aerobic or anaerobic work). During aerobic exercise the waste products are easily disposed of by the body. The limiting factors to energy production, and consequently the onset of fatigue, are the availability of glycogen and oxygen.

Training improves cardiovascular performance and oxygen delivery to the muscles but there is a finite limit to the amount of glycogen that can be stored in the body. The total stored is sufficient for about two hours of intense aerobic exercise only. If you run for more than two hours without feeding you will soon run out of fuel for your muscles. This is what is known as 'the wall' or 'the knock'.

Yet another cause, which has more to do with 'central fatigue' – the feeling of overall deep tiredness rather than just muscle ache – is related to the level of a chemical called tryptophan in the brain. Exercise increases the amount of tryptophan entering the brain, which in turn increases the level of another chemical called serotonin or 5-hydroxytryptamine. This chemical may be implicated in the condition known as subjective or perceived fatigue, in which the person feels the need for a rest. This may be a protective mechanism to prevent us having to tolerate further pain or discomfort.

WHAT IS SWEATING?

Exercise produces body heat. Long-distance runners may have body temperatures two to three degrees higher than normal. However, human beings must maintain a constant internal body temperature to function efficiently. This range is between 36°C and 38°C (97°F to 100°F). Outside these ranges, we can suffer from hyperthermia (overheating – heat cramps, heat exhaustion and heat stroke) or hypothermia (drop in body temperature – reduced heart rate, reduced respiratory rate, frost-nip and frost-bite). If the body temperature rises, we respond by sweating. As the sweat evaporates, it causes cooling. Similarly, in cold

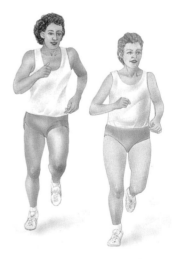

If you run for more than two hours without eating or drinking, you will soon run out of fuel for your muscles.

conditions we will shiver to generate body heat, to maintain a constant internal temperature.

The amount of sweat produced at high levels of activity can be enormous. It has been calculated that a marathon runner who completes the race in two and a half hours may lose more than five litres of fluid during that time as sweat. This is necessary to keep the body temperature from climbing, which would in turn impair the athlete's ability to function. However, if the fluid loss is too great, dehydration and heat stroke may result.

To avoid this problem, remember to:

- drink early in your exercise session

- drink small quantities

- drink frequently.

WHAT IS MUSCLE CRAMP?

Cramp is a sudden sustained and uncoordinated spasm or contraction of a muscle. It may be caused by dehydration, fatigue, muscle damage or low blood sugar levels, or a combination of these factors. To date, there has been no complete explanation for its development. Cramp often affects the hip, thigh and calf muscles during prolonged exercise. Relief can be obtained by gentle stretching and rest.

HOW ARE SPRINTERS DIFFERENT FROM MARATHON RUNNERS?

Having the right body composition can give an athlete the edge. At the highest levels of competition, it is unusual to find competitors who do not conform to the general physical attributes common to that sport – for example, most gymnasts are short, light and muscular, whereas height is an asset in basketball players.

The other significant variation is in muscle fibre type. There are two: fast twitch and slow twitch. The proportion of each in a particular muscle is inherited from your parents.

Fast twitch fibres

This type of muscle fibre reaches peak tension quickly, fatigues quickly and so uses anaerobic metabolism. Muscles with a preponderance of these fibres are powerful.

Slow twitch fibres

These have a slow contraction time, are low in power and use aerobic metabolism predominantly. These fibres predominate in the muscles of people who are good at long distance events.

Aerobic exercise such as jogging and cycling uses slow twitch fibres, whereas activities that require bursts of energy use fast twitch fibres. Marathon runners possess more than 90 per cent slow twitch fibres in their calves or thighs, whereas sprinters may have only 25 per cent. Slow twitch fibres are adapted to utilise aerobic energy, whereas fast twitch fibres use anaerobic energy stores.

HOW DOES FITNESS AFFECT THE BODY?

Generally it takes eight to ten weeks of regular training before you start to notice any benefits.

The cardiovascular system

Regular exercise changes your heart in several ways: your heart rate becomes slower, and the amount of blood the heart beat pumps (called the stroke volume) increases. The ventricles (the lower chambers in the heart) also become bigger.

These changes work in conjunction with the changes in your muscles to ensure that your body has the capacity to do more exercise before it starts to feel the effects. As it is beating more slowly, your heart has to work less hard and your blood pressure is also affected. It is lower after a work-out in normal people (those who are healthy and do not have high blood pressure), and regular work-outs make the rise in blood pressure during exercise slower and smoother. In people with mild hypertension (raised blood pressure), regular moderate exercise also reduces blood pressure by about 10 millimetres of mercury (mmHg), which is more effective than some medications.

There is also evidence that the electrical activity of the heart becomes more stable with regular exercise, so that sudden changes in heart rhythm (which sometimes lead to sudden death) are less likely.

Muscles

Although the number of muscle fibres does not increase, they become bigger and stronger. The blood supply to the muscle fibres also improves, which means that more blood and oxygen can be transported to and from the muscle than before. The enzymes that help convert energy stores to energy for muscle contraction also become more efficient. They make better use of the available oxygen supply, and produce less lactic acid, so the muscle tires less easily. Overall, the performance of the muscle improves.

Lungs

Lungs are responsible for bringing enough oxygen to the body tissues and meeting the increased demand during exercise. Although they do not change size, the amount of air they can take in and breathe out increases. Breathing rate at rest also becomes slower, which allows a comfortable increase during exercise.

Bone

Bone density is maintained and improved through exercise. Osteoporosis – the thinning of the bones that is a common cause of fractures in older people – is more severe in those individuals who have led inactive lives. Studies have demonstrated that the density of the hip bone and lower spine correlates closely with good stamina. Good bone density prevents fractures and loss of mobility later in life.

Joints and tendons

Regular movement of the joints helps to increase flexibility and prevents stiffness. The cartilage that lines the bones becomes thicker, and both ligaments and tendons become more strongly attached to bone. This, combined with stronger muscles and bones, means that exercised joints are more stable and less vulnerable to twisting and other injury.

Other changes

Exercise changes the existing pattern of blood lipids by increasing the levels of high-density lipo-proteins (HDL) and decreasing the low-density lipoprotein (LDL) level. These are both types of blood cholesterol, and it is thought that, whereas HDL protects against heart disease, LDL promotes fatty deposit formation within blood vessels which can lead to heart attacks. A favourable ratio of HDL to LDL is therefore consistent with lowered coronary heart disease risk.

The way the body deals with insulin is also altered, so that less insulin is required to deal with the blood glucose rise that happens after you've eaten. This can be beneficial for people at risk of diabetes as well as for those who already have the condition.

At maximal levels of training, the amount of oxygen in the blood increases, because the body tissues have become more efficient at extracting oxygen from the blood. The distribution of blood to active tissues also improves.

Psychological changes

People who exercise are less prone to depression and anxiety. What's more, exercise is a good outlet for feelings of stress, tension and aggression – people who exercise regularly sleep better and gain a sense of well-being. Exercise can be used to treat mild cases of anxiety and depression – in these situations it can be as helpful as drugs or psychotherapy. Severe depression or mental illness does not, however, respond to exercise.

It is still unclear why exercise has mental effects, but It is likely that somehow brain chemicals are altered. Two types of chemicals have been implicated: they are called endorphins and central monoamines, but their exact role is still unknown. They may also be responsible for 'runner's high' – the state of euphoria that some long-distance runners report.

KEY POINTS

✓ Regular exercise produces the 'training effect'

✓ Strength, speed, flexibility and endurance are the components of fitness

✓ Skill and flexibility are important in preventing injury

✓ After 8–10 weeks of regular training, benefits are noted: muscles are stronger, lungs more efficient and bones strengthened, and we feel psychologically better

All about training

TRAINING GOALS

At the most scientific level, training is all about conditioning the body so that it is tailor-made for the sport in question. This includes developing the right metabolic pathways to produce energy, the right ratio of anaerobic/aerobic fitness, the right strength in the right muscles and so on. This kind of approach is essential for the highest levels of competition, but even if you're an amateur it is worth considering specific areas to work on for your particular sport.

Non-competitive athletes may have different training goals – to lose or maintain weight, to gain muscular strength or to become fit enough for a trekking holiday, for example. All training, however, conforms to four principles.

The principle of individuality

We are all different in the way we adapt to a training programme. Therefore everyone must adopt a programme that suits them personally and takes into account their specific needs as an individual.

The principle of specificity

Training programmes are very sport specific and you would not train to be a marathon runner by practising sprinting or train for a game of golf by kicking penalty shots. Choosing the right training programme is therefore essential. Think of the programme as a 'load' that must be 'heavy' enough to increase your fitness. If the load is too light, no training effect takes place. It can be made heavier by increasing the training frequency, duration and intensity.

The principle of disuse

This may follow illness or injury. After a period of two to three weeks of non-activity (even if you have been training regularly before), your state of fitness will drop to that which meets the needs of your daily activities only. This is the principle of disuse and explains why injury can be disastrous for top athletes. It is therefore important to try to organise an alternative activity which helps you maintain some level of fitness while you recover.

The principle of progressive overload

As you become fit you find that you are able to stress your body more than when you were untrained or unfit. This is the principle of progressive overload. It involves working the body harder than normal and as you adapt you can work at a higher level.

PHASES IN TRAINING

You may not be used to the time and discipline required for a regular training programme. To begin with, get yourself accustomed to the frequency of training – say, going to the gym three times a week – until it becomes more of a habit that fits in easily with the rest of your life. Keep the duration of training and the intensity deliberately in check until this happens.

Once the habit is more established, increase the amount of time you spend working out. Finally, increase the intensity – how hard you work out. This of course is subjective, and some days the training programme will feel harder than others.

Athletes usually need to increase the frequency, duration and intensity of training for maximum fitness, but the trade-off is that the harder they train the more likely injury becomes. Adequate rest and recovery are also crucial, and so sports coaches vary the programme for athletes in terms of intensity and emphasis, so that the athlete can peak when it is necessary. Non-athletes can adopt a similar approach, so that boredom does not become a reason to stop regular exercise.

Another aspect of training is that very few sports are 'continuous' in the sense that a 100-metre sprint and a marathon are – sports such as squash, football and basketball require bursts of high energy followed by short periods of rest or less intense activity, spread over a period of, say, an hour and a half. This clearly requires a mixture of different types of fitness, and a typical training programme in these circumstances would be as shown in the box on pages 20–1.

The sports coach would ensure that these phases (which are progressive, that is, more physically demanding) blend in with the individual's mastery of the necessary technique and skills, but this gives an idea of the different elements required for high performance.

Aerobic endurance training

You need this to build up your capacity for continuous work, and it is usually a mixture of high and moderate intensity. Aerobic capacity is important in long-distance running or swimming, sports such as football or basketball where you may be running for some time, and for climbing and trekking.

Aerobic sessions should be a minimum of 30 minutes each. The heart rate (HR) should be kept constant between 130 and 160 beats per minute, that is, between 67 and 75 per cent of the maximum heart rate (MHR). These types of sessions can be applied to activities such as running and cycling. The sessions can consist of cycling or running or mixtures of each, whichever the person prefers.

Anaerobic endurance training

This kind of training develops an athlete's ability to run faster for longer distances. The energy stores are rapidly depleted as the athlete starts to run fast, so energy must be produced anaerobically and the runner quickly goes into oxygen debt. The typical duration of anaerobic training is 20 seconds to 80 seconds, that is, 150–400 metres.

Training progresses not by increasing the distance but by reducing the rest between repetitions.

Anaerobic speed training

This is what gives a sprinter the power to run at full speed for a short time. It is also useful in other sports that require short-term high intensity activity, such as the long jump, running for a catch in cricket or vaulting in gymnastics. The metabolic pathway in the body which produces energy for this kind of activity is part of the anaerobic (non-oxygen-requiring) system known as the phosphogen system (see page 9). It is quick-acting and supplies high energy for a few seconds. The energy stores are quickly depleted but can be restored rapidly with training. Sprinters commonly run at full speed for about 10 seconds, then walk back slowly for two or three minutes. In that time, their energy stores can be replaced, and they are ready to run again. Doing cycles of running and walking like this can train the body to become efficient in delivery and use of phosphogen stores, and a trained athlete can do this many times before becoming fatigued.

PATTERNS OF TRAINING

Continuous training, interval training and circuit training are all forms of aerobic training.

Continuous training

This is training at a certain level (either high or moderate intensity) for a long distance or time period, for example, jogging for five miles or using the bicycle for 45 minutes. High intensity (85 per cent maximum heart rate) is very effective for aerobic endurance training, whereas lower intensity continuous work-outs (60–70 per cent maximum heart rate) is less stressful on the heart and lungs, and suitable for people who want to maintain a certain level of fitness, or for the middle-aged person who wants to become fit.

Interval training

This involves alternate periods of intense work with periods of lower exertion or rest. It is frequently used when training for swimming, cross country or track events, and allows the athlete to achieve the greatest possible workload with the smallest physiological strain (fatigue). For example, a runner may do a 4,800-metre run alternating between a 400-metre fast interval and a 800-metre recovery interval. The whole session should last 20 to 30 minutes although élite athletes may work for up to 60 minutes. Its advantage over continuous training is that it allows the athlete to work harder for longer because of the rest periods.

Circuit training

This involves going through a series of different activities which have to be completed as quickly as possible – such as skipping, press-ups, sit-ups, running on the spot and so on. Circuit training does increase aerobic fitness, but is particularly good for increasing strength, muscle endurance and flexibility. Heart and lung fitness can be improved by running more quickly in between each station.

AN EXAMPLE OF A NON

Day	Exercise type	Pattern
Monday	Cycle or run	Steady effort
Tuesday	Circuit training	30 seconds per station
Wednesday	Recovery	Active
Thursday	Cycle or run	1 minute of effort, 1 minute for recove
Friday	Strength training	3 sets of 10 repetitions per station
Saturday	Recovery	Passive
Sunday	Cycle or run	Steady effort

All activities should be preceded and followed by at least a five-minute war

HOW TO DEVELOP STRENGTH

You can train with the specific aim of increasing your strength. This approach used to be called 'weight training' but is now known as 'resistance training' because muscle is developed by working against some form of resistance. Various types of resistance can be used.

Free weights (barbells, dumbbells, etc.)

These are still very popular. Different exercises can be prescribed to strengthen different muscle groups. One drawback is that free weights can be lifted only in the vertical plane (that is, up and down against gravity) and this is not always easy to convert to sports that may require movement in other directions.

The classic system of weight training was designed in the 1940s, based on the concept of 'repetition maximum' or RM. A 10-RM load was what an athlete could lift ten times before fatigue stopped him doing the next lift; a 5-RM could be lifted five times, and so on.

SPECIFIC TRAINING SCHEDULE

Effort	Duration	Type of activity
70%	1 hour	Aerobic endurance
75%	30 minutes	Aerobic speed
<50%	30 minutes	Aerobic
60–80%	40 minutes	Anaerobic endurance
70–90%	1 hour	Anaerobic speed
NA	NA	NA
65%	2 hours	Aerobic endurance

/down routine (see pages 30–3).   NA, not applicable.

Therefore a 1-RM load was heaviest, and could be lifted only once. How heavy each RM was varied from person to person.

A traditional programme would be:

- 10 repetitions with 0.5 of a 10-RM load

- 10 repetitions with 0.75 of a 10-RM load

- 10 repetitions with a 10-RM load.

Training should take place three times weekly and strength should

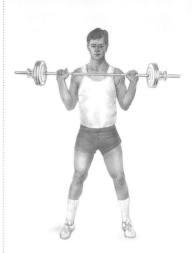

Barbell with variable disc weights at either end.

improve measurably in five weeks.

Experienced lifters still find this system useful, but now often use 5- to 7-RM weights and work out five times a week – so moving towards more intense work-outs. Stacked weights with pulley systems have replaced free weights in many areas; they have the advantage of being safer, and also can be designed to allow for movement in different directions.

Isometrics

Isometric contraction means contracting a muscle without movement, for example, pushing an arm against a fixed weight like a brick wall. This is now no longer in favour, because static muscle contraction is not a feature in many sports. Strength gains tend to be

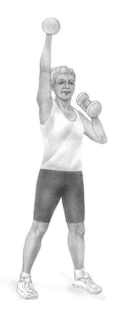

Dumb-bells.

limited to the limb position used in training.

Isokinetics and variable resistance systems

These are the commercially available systems seen in larger gyms, which produce resistance by hydraulics, compressed air, flywheels and the like. They are designed to produce resistance of a pre-set constant velocity, or to match the ability of the athlete to apply forces throughout a range of movement. They are very specific and can load a muscle group continuously through a range of movement, but the drawback is that strength gained at one velocity may not transfer to another velocity, and many sports require acceleration of movement, which cannot be trained with isokinetics. Many machines are required to meet all an athlete's needs.

Body weight

Body weight can be used as a form of resistance, as in jumping or running uphill. This is particularly good for developing the explosive

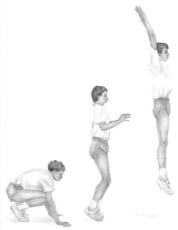

Body weight is a useful form of resistance.

strength needed for some sports. Plyometrics is a system of 'depth-jumping' and consists of body weight exercises. They require intense effort on each push-off and emphasise minimal time spent on the ground and maximum height in the air. Roughly defined, plyometrics is a collection of jumps, hops, leaps and bounds performed with speed and intensity. Plyometrics exercises

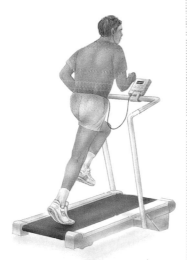

There are many variable resistance exercise machines, which exercise a wide variety of muscle groups.

are the link between strength and speed.

Skill-specific resistance

These include special contraptions such as rubber tubing to resist golf swings and tennis serves. Runners and swimmers can tow a heavy object, or wear weights or drag suits to increase their strength in the context of their sport. The drawback is that sometimes this kind of training can interfere with the normal muscular response – for instance, strapping weights to a runner's ankles makes the legs work differently from when he or she is running without them.

REST, RECOVERY AND DETRAINING

Rest and recovery are very important components of any training schedule. Overtraining leads to a tendency to chronic fatigue and physical breakdown, and makes an athlete more vulnerable to injury and strain. This of course is the dilemma for top athletes, because once they ease up on training all the adaptations they have acquired start to reverse. Many are tempted to return to training too soon after injury or illness.

The skilful coach will take rest and recovery into serious consideration when designing a programme, to ensure that the athlete peaks at the right time.

Athletes should have one full rest day per week and one day of active recovery. This should take the form of light rhythmical activities such as jogging or swimming and should follow a day of hard training or competition.

Detraining is a phenomenon by which the physiological benefits of training are lost because of

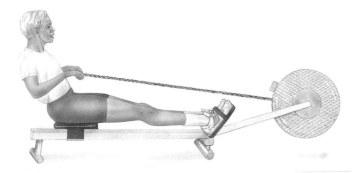

Exercise equipment can simulate closely the particular characteristics of specific sports.

prolonged inactivity through injury or change in lifestyle. It becomes significant after periods of at least 14 days in trained Individuals.

Tips for beginners

Regular exercise and sport have become increasingly popular among non-athletes of all ages, who participate for the sake of their health and well-being rather than competitively. They can be as highly trained as athletes, but may not want to spend the time and effort required for peak fitness. You are likely to get different advice from different people on how best to do this. Generally, however, It is agreed that a balanced programme with aerobic work at its core is the best approach. You also need to spend time on flexibility, relaxation and strength work.

The first question anyone unused to exercise should ask is: am I fit enough to start exercising? It you have had any episodes of unexplained dizziness or fainting or chest pains, heart trouble or high blood pressure or are already suffering from a condition such as diabetes, asthma or chronic chest disease, it is important to consult your own GP before starting any activity.

The key to success is gentle steady progress. Children should ideally be introduced to a sport as early as possible and be given realistic goals and opportunities for success to encourage them to stay involved. Most children are introduced to a sport such as swimming by parents, whereas more complex sports such as team games may be led by a PE instructor or teacher. Older children will naturally develop their own interests, preferences and motivation, all of which are important and become important factors, but body size may also influence their choice of sport.

People in mid-life and older age groups may decide to take up a particular activity through the Influence of friends or colleagues or because a recent illness has given them the incentive to lose weight and become active. The age factor is very important and the earlier a person is introduced to a sport or activity the better his or her performance is likely to be.

Whatever your age, however, there is no point in exercising madly for two or three weeks only to find that you can't continue because you have overdone it. One good way to start is to build exercise around your everyday routine so that it becomes part of your lifestyle. There are many ways of doing this but you could try:

- walking to work if possible or getting off the bus a stop or two earlier

- using the stairs instead of the lift

- walking to the shops or post box

- parking the car a mile from work and walking the rest of the way

- walking the dog (or take walks around the block three times a day, if you do not have one to walk)

- going on cycle runs (for shopping and other errands) or cycle rides

- organising family walks.

You need to take exercise three times a week for at least 20 minutes before you start to gain any benefit. A reasonable 'maintenance' level would be, say, moderate exercise for 30 minutes, three times a week. As mentioned above, you should get used to exercising frequently before you increase the duration and finally the intensity. For the non-athlete it does not matter if progress is a little slow, but each step should be made over eight- to ten-week periods.

If you are overweight or you have not engaged in physical activity for several years, consider non-weight-bearing forms of exercise such as swimming or cycling. This reduces the risk of injuring your knees, feet and ankles which may otherwise object to the new demands being placed upon them. After several months, improvements in cardiorespiratory (heart–lung) and aerobic efficiency can be measured and you may also have lost weight.

HOW HARD AM I EXERCISING?

How should you go about estimating how hard a work-out is? Some gyms use a subjective scale – starting with light, then moderate, severe and very severe. Moderate exercise is exercise that requires effort, but which can be maintained for about 20 minutes without severe exhaustion. This level is suitable for non-athletes. Another approach uses pulse counting.

Calorie counting

This is another way to assess the intensity of exercise. The more calories used up during exercise, the more energy is used, and the greater the intensity of exercise.

Energy used is normally expressed as kilocalories per minute (kcal/min). One kilocalorie is 1,000 calories. Many exercise machines allow you to monitor your calorific output.

The energy used during various activities has been calculated for average-sized people. Some examples are shown in the box.

Clearly, in a 30-minute work-

CALORIE COUNTING

Activity	Energy used (in kcal/min)
Walking	
average pace	4
fast	6
Cricket	6
Dancing	6
Cycling	7
Keep fit class	8
Swimming	8
Tennis, badminton	8
Football	10
Squash	13
Running	13

out, the more calories you use, the harder you are exercising. For a moderate work-out, you should aim to burn between 250 and 300 kilocalories.

ASSESSING IMPROVEMENTS IN FITNESS

Again, one of the simplest methods is simply to count your pulse rate. If you are in your twenties it should be approximately 60 beats per minute, and as you get older this resting pulse rate will rise and it will be around 80 to 90 beats per minute as you reach retirement. With all forms of regular training and activity this resting pulse rate will reduce.

Another method of assessing fitness is to measure your pulse rate during exercise and then stop exercising and note how quickly it returns to normal. Even after vigorous activity the pulse rate with training will come back to normal within 10 to 15 minutes. If you note this over a period of time in relation to the type of activity you have

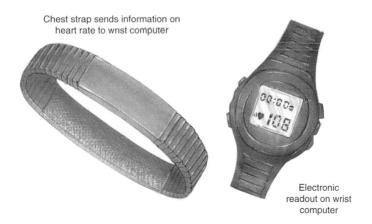

Chest strap sends information on heart rate to wrist computer

Electronic readout on wrist computer

An electronic heart monitor will tell you how hard you are exercising.

PULSE COUNTING

This is a way of assessing your fitness and also working out your maximum heart rate. Most authorities now agree that the maximum heart rate is calculated as follows:

220 − Age = Maximum heart rate.

This can then be used to calculate training intensities.

Feel your pulse on the front of your wrist just above the skin creases near the thumb edge of the forearm and count it for one minute. This is called your 'resting pulse rate'.

The increase in pulse rate that you must achieve to improve the function of your cardiovascular system, which services your muscles, is called 'the loading pulse rate' and can be calculated by the following formula:

$$\text{Loading} = \text{Resting pulse} + \frac{60}{100} \left(220 - \text{Age} - \text{Resting pulse}\right)$$

For example, if you are 35 years old with a resting pulse rate of 60 beats per minute (bpm) you have to increase your pulse above the resting pulse rate by 75 beats per minute (that is, 135 beats per minute in total):

Loading pulse rate = 60 + 60% × (220 − 35 − 60)
$$= 60 + 60\% \times 125$$
$$= 60 + 75$$
Loading pulse rate = 135 beats per minute.

Therefore you must aim for a pulse rate of 135 beats per minute to be maintained for at least 20 to 30 minutes per session of activity. This is your loading pulse rate. Using this principle you need only a watch with a second hand to improve your fitness. It is unwise to be too dogmatic about workloads and duration and intensity of training for non-athletes, because the maximum heart rate can vary quite remarkably from one person to another of the same age. Nevertheless, regular gentle aerobic exercise combined with flexibility, relaxation and strength exercises should be part of most people's lives.

been doing (that is, how long did it take you to cover a fixed distance while running or walking?), you will have a record of all your results and be able to see the improvements in your fitness with training.

FLEXIBILITY

Why stretch?

Stretching helps to increase the range of movement in joints or a group of joints. It reduces muscle tension, helps to prevent muscle strains and allows the body to relax. It also prepares the body for activity; by focusing on each group of muscles as you stretch you develop body awareness. There is also some suggestion that regular stretching exercises help promote circulation to the areas focused upon.

Stretching done correctly should not be painful

As you stretch, relax and focus your attention on the muscle or group of muscles you are working on. It takes time to loosen tight muscles but becomes easier as you progress. Stretch until you feel a slight tension in the muscle, hold this for 15–20 seconds and the tension will ease slightly. Breathing should be normal, breathe out as you stretch, hold the stretch as you breathe in, then stretch a little further as you breathe out again. DO NOT HOLD YOUR BREATH.

Make sure that you wear loose and comfortable clothing.

The wrong way

Never bounce as you stretch or stretch to a point where it becomes painful. If the stretch interferes with breathing, relax, ease off, breathe normally and begin again.

After the first easy stretching exercises and some light exercises to warm the muscles up, you should restretch until you feel mild tension within the muscles. Regular stretching exercises improve flexibility.

SPECIFIC TRAINING PROGRAMMES FOR DIFFERENT GOALS

Training can be adapted to individual requirements and will involve combinations of aerobic/anaerobic work with or without resistance training. If you have a specific goal in mind, ask for advice from the trainer at the local gym or club and also get advice on the right kind of diet (see 'Useful addresses, page 94).

OVERTRAINING

Training is all about achieving increasing fitness without paying the price of increasing injury. Training too intensively can lead to physical exhaustion. Tired muscles do not perform well, and are more liable to strains. Nor do they hold

STRETCHING

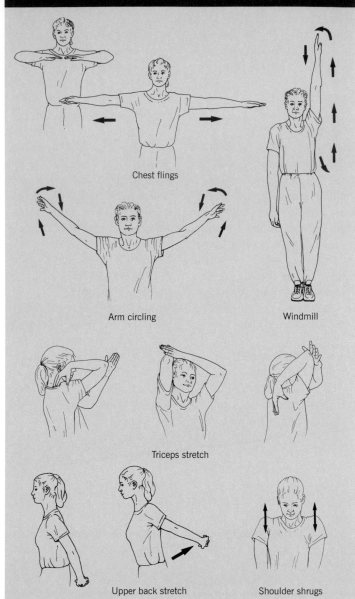

Chest flings

Windmill

Arm circling

Triceps stretch

Upper back stretch

Shoulder shrugs

STRETCHING

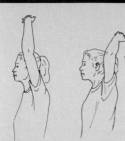
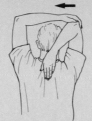
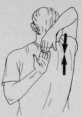

Above head shoulder stretch

Bent arm shoulder stretch

Shoulder stretch

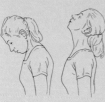

Neck stretches

Side bends

Torso stretch

Trunk turns

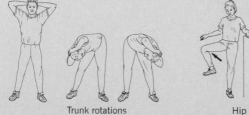

Trunk rotations

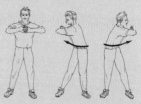

Hip rotation

STRETCHING

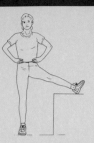

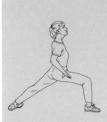

Groin stretch

Side stretch

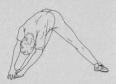

Abductors stretch 1

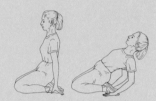

Sitting quadriceps stretch

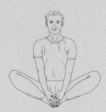

Abductors stretch 2

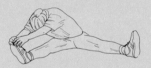

Hamstring stretch

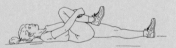

Alternative hamstring stretch

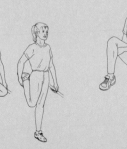

Quadriceps stretch

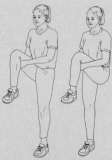

Gluteal stretch

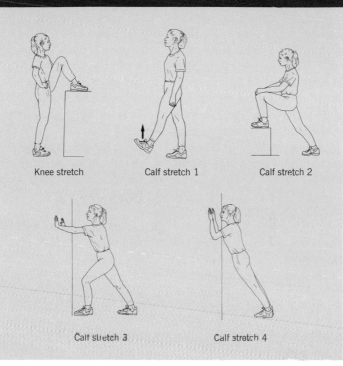

Knee stretch

Calf stretch 1

Calf stretch 2

Calf stretch 3

Calf stretch 4

the limbs tightly, and falls, sprains and fractures may occur because of muscular exhaustion. Fatigue leads to poor balance and coordination, and this can lead to more injury. Adequate rest after exercise is crucial to allow the body to restore its energy, and repair the 'wear and tear' that goes with exercise.

Prolonged exertion can put repeated stress on certain bones and actually cause small fractures. One example of this is the so-called 'march fracture' of the foot, which is commonly seen in marching soldiers and runners. These fractures cause pain and swelling, but may not be easy to see on an X-ray till later, when they leave a callus (new bone growth around the fracture) on healing.

In the long run, joints that are over-used through sport are more prone to osteoarthritis as the person gets older. For instance, skiers put a lot of strain on their knees for long periods of time, and many have damage to the cartilage of their knees, which are worn down through over-use. In later years this may lead to stiffness and pain on walking. Runners may also have problems with their knees and ankles later on. The risk of such long-term injury has led to interest in exercise regimens that do not cause any joint damage. Examples of these are low-impact aerobics, swimming, water aerobics and resistance training using stretch bands.

WARM UP, COOL DOWN

The warm-up
Warm-up reduces the risk of injury and improves your performance by increasing the speed and force of muscular contraction and, when it is related to the particular activity you're about to undertake, it seems to sharpen coordination and improve rhythm. Although its mechanisms are poorly understood, it seems to permit faster adaptation to the activity and brings on so-called 'second wind' more readily.

When warming up:

- The activity should be intense enough to make you perspire but not so intense that it causes fatigue.

- Include loosening and stretching exercises.

- Include movements that mirror the activity you're about to begin; for example, gentle

A SIMPLE WARM-UP ROUTINE

Duration   10 to 15 minutes

Objective   To increase the body temperature and prepare the body physiologically for exercise

Components

1. Pulse raiser: five-minute jog to increase the heart rate and make the body sweat

2. Static stretching to reduce the risk of muscular injury – five minutes

3. Sports-specific warm-up – five minutes replicating the event that you will do, for example, practising your swing before teeing off for a round of golf

jogging and stretching before a run and swinging a golf club or hitting some practice shots before a game of golf.

- Taper off your warm-up so that it ends about five minutes before you start your activity, to allow yourself to recover from any slight fatigue.

- Keeping warm after warming up is important, so make sure you're appropriately dressed.

The cool-down

A cool-down must be done at a much lower intensity than the preceding exercise and should last about five to ten minutes. Check your pulse rate at the end of exercise and again at the end of the cool-down. It should be within 20 beats of the normal resting pulse rate. At the end of the exercise period jog for five minutes keeping to a walk, then carry out long, slow, sustained stretches of the major muscle groups such as the quadriceps, hamstrings, calf muscles and pectoral girdle. Make sure you wear extra comfortable clothing to prevent over-cooling.

STIFFNESS AND SORENESS

Muscle soreness can be divided into two types. Acute muscle soreness occurs towards the end of exercise or immediately afterwards. It is the result of the accumulation of lactic acid or hydrogen ions in the muscle, which makes it more acidic and less efficient. Activity also shifts more blood into the muscle, which leads to the 'pumped up' feeling that people experience after weights or prolonged endurance training. This kind of muscle soreness disappears soon after the exercise has stopped.

Delayed onset soreness comes on a day or two after exercise. It seems to be caused by actual muscle damage. When looked at under a microscope, there are signs of inflammation in the muscle. This type of soreness is associated with a different type of muscle contraction called eccentric contraction, which occurs especially after walking or running down hill, and disappears after several days of rest.

If it is very severe, taking simple pain-killers such as aspirin and ibuprofen will help. If you do experience muscle soreness then gentle rhythmical activities will ease the pain, such as slow jogging and swimming. It is important that the intensity should be dramatically decreased.

To prevent soreness, start training at low intensity and take your time to progress over the first few weeks. Avoid running straight downhill to ensure that you do not suffer eccentric contraction.

Massage, heat and Radox baths

will help ease pain. A good cool-down also helps to reduce post-exercise soreness because it reduces metabolic poisoning levels of lactate within the muscle groups.

WHY DO PEOPLE DIE SUDDENLY DURING EXERCISE?

We have all heard stories of people who died suddenly during a game of squash or while out jogging. The primary cause of these sudden deaths is a heart rhythm disturbance called ventricular fibrillation. Many people who die in this way have some risk factor for heart disease – they may be obese, unused to exercise or have had previous bouts of chest pain. Some do not give any clues in their medical history.

Sports such as squash are extremely vigorous, and someone who is just starting to play it may be unused to the level of exertion required. The excitement of the game may also distract a person from noticing the exertion till they are truly exhausted or it is too late. It has been said that 'one should get fit to play squash rather than play squash to get fit'. The stress that such exertion poses on the body releases certain hormones which may play a part in heart rhythm disturbance.

Anyone who has a history of cardiac problems, or is obese or unused to exercise, should get a doctor's advice before starting an exercise programme. Take it slowly and gently, and start with the gentler activities such as walking and swimming. Listen to your body and stop when you feel any chest pain, dizziness or faintness.

KEY POINTS

✓ A typical non-specific programme (for all-round fitness) should include combinations of aerobic and anaerobic activities

✓ Use calorie counting to assess the intensity of your exercise

✓ Pulse counting is valuable to assess fitness and to work out your maximum heart rate

✓ Warm up and cool down to reduce the risk of injury and to improve performance

When extra care is needed

CHILDREN

Children call exercising 'going out to play' and their hearts, lungs, muscles and joints respond very positively. When it comes to taking part in training sessions for those children and adolescents who are seriously interested in a particular sport, however, care is needed to avoid repetitive stresses on their growing bones, muscles and tendons. Overtraining and undue repetitive stresses can lead to problems with the shoulders and elbows, knees and heels. One important point to remember is that, because they are growing fast, shoes, gumshields and helmets will need to be regularly refitted and replaced. Up to the age of 14, boys and girls show similar injury patterns but, after that, boys are three times more likely to be injured than girls of the same age.

If you're looking after children who are exercising outside, bear in mind that they are more susceptible to heat- and cold-induced illness and injury than adults so you need to be extra careful in very hot or cold weather.

Children can also undertake standard training programmes. For example, they can begin resistance training from the age of seven provided that they are sensibly introduced to basic exercises with little or no weight. Over the years the number of exercises can be gradually increased until around the age of 16 or older when the child progresses to an adult-type resistance training programme. Any such programme must always be properly supervised by someone who knows what they're doing. Children can improve their strength with resistance training with little or no change in muscle size.

Children also respond positively to anaerobic training which increases their capacity to use this kind of energy and to aerobic training to build up their endurance. Regular training reduces their total body fat without affecting their growth or the rate at which they mature. The most important thing is to avoid overtraining.

WOMEN

Women experience the same training effects as men but in general tend to lose less fat. They respond extremely well to strength training, becoming stronger and more powerful without necessarily increasing muscle bulk. Their heart and lungs adapt in much the same way as men's. They develop a greater capacity to deliver oxygen efficiently to their tissues with endurance training.

If you're a woman taking part in activities that involve rhythmic repetitive movements, such as long-distance running or aerobics, always wear a well-fitting sports bra or apply grease to your nipples to prevent chafing. As adolescent girls develop into women, the alignment of the thighs and the pelvis changes and as a result women are more prone to knee and ankle injuries than men. Get medical advice if you develop persistent knee problems or pain in the ankles.

There is no reason why you shouldn't continue doing your usual exercise or sport while you're having your period, although some women

athletes prefer to regulate their periods by going on the pill. Some types of activity may result in irregular periods and decreased fertility and, when training is intense, periods may stop completely because of a fall in the level of the female hormone oestrogen. This is of no consequence in the short term, especially if having a child is not an issue, but, if it continues for several years, the low levels of oestrogen put the woman at risk of developing osteoporosis.

Women who experience severe symptoms of PMS (premenstrual syndrome) may have problems in sports where fine judgement is required. Not everyone is affected and those who are may find regular exercise helps to alleviate the problem, and it can also ease painful periods. Very heavy periods can interfere with exercise and, in severe cases, can cause anaemia which makes you feel very tired. A poor diet may also result in anaemia, but, whatever the cause, the condition needs to be diagnosed and treated by your doctor.

Exercise during pregnancy

When you are pregnant, your body undergoes a series of dramatic changes. Your weight increases by about 25 per cent and your metabolic rate and oxygen consumption increase as well. You need 3,000 more kilocalories per day.

The thyroid gland enlarges in 70 per cent of women and there are changes in carbohydrate metabolism, plasma proteins and nitrogen balance.

The volume of blood circulating round your body increases by up to 40 per cent, and its composition changes too, with higher levels of red blood cells and blood fats (lipids). Your blood also clots more easily. Your heart rate rises as does the stroke/volume of the heart (the amount of blood pumped into the circulation with each beat of the heart). You'll notice a difference in the way your bowels and bladder work, and the ureters (tubes) leading from the kidneys to the bladder expand.

You don't need to stop exercising during pregnancy. Indeed there is good evidence that regular exercise may improve the quality of the pregnancy and make your contractions more effective during labour. There are, however, some types of exercise that you should avoid while you're pregnant (see page 40) and you'll need to reduce the amount you do in the last three months.

If you have been exercising before becoming pregnant you should carry on but reduce the intensity of the exercise with a recommended maximum heart rate of 140 beats per minute. Don't do more than 15 minutes at a time two to three times per week. If you did not exercise before your pregnancy began, be careful about taking it up now and get advice from your doctor, midwife or antenatal teacher.

Taking the right kind of exercise in pregnancy offers a range of beneficial effects. It is good for your:

- bowel function

- self-image

- psychological state

- weight control

- muscle tone

- joint flexibility.

Every woman needs to have her own, personalised exercise programme which will include a planned tailing off as her pregnancy advances. Remember to take increased rest periods and keep your maximum effort down to 50 to 60 per cent of your pre-pregnancy levels.

During your pregnancy, avoid any movements that involve severe flexion or hyperextension of the trunk (bending forwards or backwards), or any breath-holding procedures such as the Valsalva manoeuvre which involves taking a deep breath and then straining

EXERCISE IN PREGNANCY

Recommended in moderation	Not recommended
Swimming	Impact aerobics (high or low)
Walking	Hang gliding
Cycling	Skiing
Isometrics	Other impact sports
	All contact sports
	Motor cycling
	Scuba diving

against a closed glottis (windpipe) as a weightlifter does when lifting a heavy weight.

Overdoing exercise or doing the wrong kind can have an adverse effect on both you and your unborn baby and slow down your baby's growth rate (intrauterine growth retardation) so that he or she weighs less than normal at birth. If you develop any symptoms while exercising, such as fainting, vaginal bleeding or chest or abdominal pain, tell your doctor or midwife immediately. You should also watch out for other possible side effects of too much exercise, such as nausea, fluid retention, headaches, painful joints and premature rupture of the membranes.

After the birth

If you feel up to it, you can start gentle exercise about four to six weeks after having your baby or around the time that the postnatal vaginal bleeding stops. You'll need to wear a good supporting nursing bra if you're breast-feeding to relieve discomfort during exercise activity.

Get expert advice on the right kind of programme to follow because breast-feeding mothers can produce increased amounts of lactic acid which is not good for the baby. Walking or swimming helps restore abdominal muscle tone and helps you get back your pre-pregnancy figure.

OLDER PEOPLE

The golden rule is to begin exercising slowly and to build up gradually. Before you start, however, it is important to visit your doctor for a check-up as a precaution. You may be advised to diet to lose weight, particularly if you are more than ten per cent over your ideal weight. It would also be appropriate to have your blood pressure, pulse rate, heart and lungs tested as well as your urine and blood. Ideal exercise for older people includes swimming, walking, golf, gentle orienteering and other aerobic activities.

KEY POINTS

✓ Avoid repetitive stresses on growing bones, muscles and tendons of children

✓ Children are more susceptible to heat- and cold-induced illness

✓ Women should wear well-fitting sports bras and/or apply grease to the nipples to prevent chafing

✓ Regular exercise in pregnancy improves the quality of contractions in labour

✓ Older people should build up exercise slowly and have a precautionary check-up before starting an exercise programme

Diet in sport and exercise

Diet and athletic performance have always been linked. You only need to scan sports magazines to see articles and advertisements recommending various foodstuffs guaranteed to help you achieve your sporting ambitions. The promises are unlimited, so it is not surprising if you end up feeling confused about what to eat and when.

It is important to enjoy your food, and healthy eating may not mean changing your eating habits dramatically. However, it may mean substituting or trying out different types of food. When you're taking regular exercise or are in training, you should eat normally but add extra calories to replace the energy you're using, unless you are trying to lose weight.

You need to make sure you have sufficient carbohydrates, proteins and fats. You'll get most (and probably all) of the vitamins and minerals you need from your food, although many people take supplements. This does no harm except in relation to vitamin A where excess intake can be toxic.

HOW MANY MEALS?

Your aim is to eat enough to sustain or even slightly exceed your output of energy. Many experts now feel that having frequent small meals improves your athletic performance but this can sometimes be difficult in practice. We suggest therefore that you eat at least three good meals a day, breakfast being particularly important. Although eating more of any kind of food will provide the extra fuel you need to compensate for the extra energy you're expending, increasing your carbohydrate intake is the ideal approach.

THE THREE MAIN FOODS

Food is used as fuel to supply

WE NEED SIX ESSENTIAL NUTRIENTS

Proteins ⎫
Carbohydrates ⎬ three main foods
Fats ⎭
Minerals
Vitamins
Water

energy and as building material for the repair and growth of tissues. We need minerals, vitamins and water in addition to proteins, carbohydrates and fats.

All foods contain one or more of these six essentials. The body-building foods are proteins, water and minerals. The energy-producers are carbohydrates and fats. Vitamins and minerals help to make these processes of building body and energy production happen efficiently.

Some athletes, especially those living on their own, do not follow a well-balanced diet so, if you notice that your performance is dropping off, take a look at your eating habits.

Carbohydrates

Carbohydrates are your main source of energy. When they are combined with oxygen (oxidised) in cells, carbon dioxide and water are formed and energy is released:

Glucose + Oxygen = Energy + Carbon dioxide + Water.

Carbohydrates are classified by nutritionists as sugars, starches and fibre.

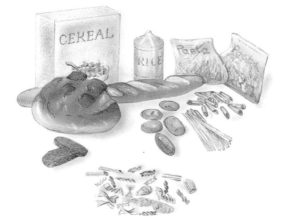

Common sources of carbohydrates include bread, cereals, pasta and potatoes.

- **Sugars:** Sugars are important sources of dietary energy. Glucose is used as fuel by your body's cells, and your brain is almost entirely dependent on it for all its functions, including thinking and growth.

Excess sugars are stored in your liver as glycogen. These stores are mobilised if you're not getting enough energy from your diet or if energy is needed quickly for exercise. If these stores are full, sugars are converted into fat and stored in adipose tissue.

- **Starches:** Starchy foods are an important part of your diet. In some parts of the world, starch provides up to 80 per cent of the total energy intake. In the UK, starch provides about 24 per cent of the total energy intake.

Raw starch is very difficult to digest. Processing, such as cooking, can change the patterns of starch molecules, making it more digestible. Heating starch in water causes it to swell and thicken. This allows it to be broken down by the digestive enzyme amylase into glucose, which can be absorbed into your body.

In the UK, the major sources of starches in the diet are staple foods such as potatoes, cereal grains (wheat, barley, maize, oats and rye) and rice.

- **Fibre:** Fibre is the major component of plant cell walls and is resistant to enzymes that digest food. Most of the fibre in the diet comes from fruit, vegetables and cereals. In wheat, maize and rice, the fibre is mainly insoluble, whereas in oats, barley and rye it is mainly soluble. In fruit and vegetables, the ratio of insoluble to soluble fibre is variable. Each kind of fibre plays a different role in digestion.

Insoluble fibre increases the bulk and wetness of faeces. It therefore prevents and relieves constipation

SOLUBLE AND INSOLUBLE FIBRE SOURCES

Soluble fibre
Beans, for example, baked
  beans
Lentils
Peas
Oats
Oranges
Apples

Insoluble fibre
Wholemeal bread
Wholemeal breakfast cereals
Wholemeal biscuits and crisp
  breads
Brown rice
Wheat bran
Oats

by holding water in your bowel. The increased bulk speeds up the transit time of faeces and reduces the pressure in your bowel.

Soluble fibre has little effect on stool bulk. However, it binds bile acids, which are rich in cholesterol. The cholesterol found in bile is usually reabsorbed into your body. Soluble fibre prevents this re-absorption so more cholesterol is lost in the faeces and less is taken back into your bloodstream. This can be important in the prevention of coronary heart disease.

The digestion and absorption of carbohydrates are slower if there is a good supply of fibre in your diet. This results in a more gradual release of glucose into your blood, which is especially important for people with diabetes. Fibre makes you feel full because once it has absorbed water it has a larger bulk.

Proteins

Proteins are used mainly for building new tissue. This might make you think that increasing the amount of protein in your diet would increase your muscle size. However, extra protein in the diet is usually unnecessary because, if it exceeds 15 to 20 per cent of your dietary intake, you simply excrete it. You should aim to take protein in the form of lean meat, fish and other protein alternatives and to eat two portions of fish per week – especially oily fish, such as sardines and mackerel.

Fats

These are the energy storehouse of the body. The average 70-kilogram (kg) person has 10.5 kg of fat (15 per cent of body weight). However, in a highly trained athlete only around 5 to 10 per cent of the body

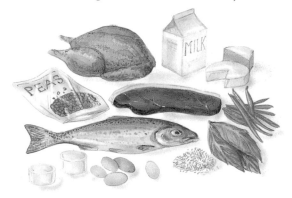

Protein can be found in animal produce and in plant foods such as cereals, beans and pulses. It is important to eat protein from a mixture of sources to ensure that you have an adequate supply of all essential amino acids.

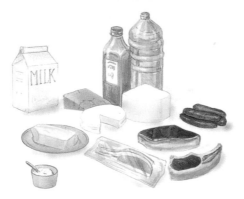

Fats in your diet come from both animal and vegetable sources and are often divided into two types: visible fat that can be seen, and invisible fat that is incorporated during cooking or manufacture.

weight will be fat. About one-fifth of dietary intake should be fat, with more coming from vegetable rather than animal sources.

Low-fat milk and other dairy foods are a good source of calcium but you should avoid eating foods that contain excessive amounts of fat or refined sugar.

Vitamins

Athletes are sometimes said to need more vitamins than other people, but there is no conclusive evidence that this is the case. Vitamins are essential for normal health, but they cannot be used as fuel. They are present in small quantities in most foods.

People who have a healthy diet are unlikely to require vitamin supplements.

- **Vitamin B$_{15}$:** Vitamin B$_{15}$ or

VITAMIN FOOD SOURCES

Vitamin A	Carrots, green vegetables
Vitamin B complex	Yeast, cereals, vegetables, fruit, milk, meats
Vitamin C	Citrus fruits, blackcurrants, green peppers, potatoes
Vitamin D	Cod liver oil, halibut oil
Vitamin E	Vegetable oil
Vitamin K	Green vegetables, liver

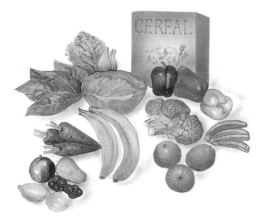

Fruit and vegetables are excellent sources of vitamins and other essential nutrients.

pangamic acid is known as one of the 'super-vitamins', and some athletes believe it to be the missing ingredient in their performance. It is dangerous. Toxic reactions to it have occurred, and one of its chemical constituents combines with saliva to form a carcinogen – a chemical that can lead to cancer formation. It is to be avoided at all costs.

Minerals

Lack of minerals can produce a range of symptoms from nausea and vomiting to extreme muscular weakness.

* **Sodium:** Sodium is obtained from animal foods and cooking salt. It becomes depleted during heavy sweating or in a humid atmosphere, and losing too much causes fatigue and muscular cramps. Tennis players

are especially at risk and you will have seen the professionals take salt tablets between games. However, unless you sweat profusely over a very long period (more than an hour), usually in a hot environment, depletion is unlikely.

* **Calcium:** This is the most common mineral in the body and an important constituent of bones and teeth. Apart from this, it also has a vital role in the clotting of the blood and in controlling the action of the heart and the muscles. It is found in milk, cheese and hard water and, if you have a healthy diet and regular exercise, you shouldn't experience a deficiency, which leads to rickets in children and thinning of the bones (osteoporosis) in adults.

* **Iron:** This is derived from eggs, meat, green vegetables and fish.

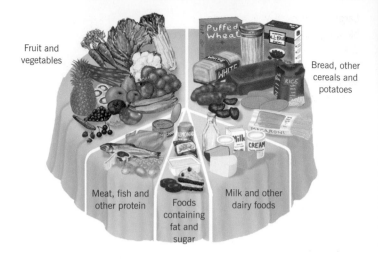

Aim to balance your intake of the different food types into the approximate proportions shown above.

Liver also has a very high iron content. It is important in the oxygen-carrying capacity of the blood and deficiency of iron leads to anaemia. This, in turn, leads to fatigue and poor physical performance. Women especially need to watch their iron intake because they lose iron through menstruation each month. They need 12 to 15 grams daily, which they may not get from an adequate diet. Many women athletes are training with anaemia. A simple blood test can check this out and, if iron supplementation fails to correct anaemia, further investigations are necessary.

Water

Around 70 per cent of our body weight is made up of water. In endurance events, such as cycling, marathons or tennis, fluid loss can be very significant, and as much as eight per cent of body weight may be lost as sweat. Dehydration is poorly tolerated by the body: it overheats, the heart rate climbs and heat exhaustion results.

When fluid is lost as sweat, more pure water than minerals is lost, and so it is more important to replace the water than the minerals. Mineral loss occurs only in extreme cases. The temperature and quantity of the water can affect how quickly it is absorbed into the body – 150 to 180 millilitres of cold water taken three to four times every hour is more cooling than warm water because it is more easily absorbed.

Large volumes of water can cause bloating and breathing discomfort. Contrary to popular myth there is no evidence that cold water causes stomach cramps – although large volumes of it may.

There is no evidence that water on its own is more easily absorbed than a mixture, for example, a cordial, but isotonic fluids which have the same tenacity as body fluids are far more easily absorbed into the digestive system and therefore are more efficient in replacing fluid loss during long periods of exercise than water alone.

TRAINING DIETS

Losing weight
Weight restriction is an integral part of certain sports, such as horse racing and boxing. Many athletes fast or dehydrate their bodies just to make the required weight. They use diuretics to increase their water loss through the urine, but dehydration leads to poor muscle strength and increased heart rate for the same amount of work – the opposite of what training is all about. If the athlete is still growing, this kind of restriction can lead to growth stunting.

If your sport requires you to be at a particular weight, you need to determine this early in the season, then work towards it gradually over four weeks or more, by controlling

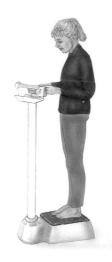

what you eat and increasing the amount of training you do.

Gaining weight
The aim here is to increase weight by increasing muscle mass. You can do this by eating more – add two or three high-carbohydrate, low-fat snacks per day. Muscle can be laid down by weight training.

The traditional body builders' diet of egg whites and chicken (that is, high protein) is a fallacy. The most efficient way to increase muscle is to train more and the body needs carbohydrate to do this. Although you need to increase your protein intake slightly, this increase should not exceed one gram per kilogram of body weight per day.

Carbohydrate or glycogen loading
This is a dietary technique to help

endurance athletes build up muscle energy stores. Although it does improve performance, it may be dangerous for older athletes (see below).

First, existing muscle stores should be depleted by taking moderately heavy exercise while not eating enough carbohydrate foods to replace what is used. This should last for two or three days; then for two or three days before the race the athlete switches to a low-exercise regime and a diet with a high carbohydrate content. The theory is that the depleted cells then super-compensate and store even greater amounts of glycogen. Less water is required during the race, but the high carbohydrate diet

SIMPLE DIETARY GUIDELINES

- Try out lots of different foods and introduce changes that fit in with your lifestyle

- Try out new recipes

- Eat foods rich in carbohydrate and fibre, but bear in mind that you may have to pay a price for a high-fibre diet: more frequent visits to the toilet and sometimes the excessive passage of wind which may be socially unacceptable, so go steadily

- Whatever changes you're making to your diet, try to make sure you still enjoy your food, and make simple changes in your eating habits that fit in with the limits of your budget and your lifestyle

- Avoid eating too many fatty and sugary foods

- Ensure that your diet provides adequate amounts of vitamins and minerals

- Don't drink too much alcohol (28 units per week for a man and 21 units per week for a woman; one unit is equivalent to half a pint of beer, a measure of spirits or a small glass of wine) and the water retention that occurs may be dangerous for middle-aged and older people. Eating huge meals can also cause heart problems in susceptible individuals. Finally, this method is probably only effective in people who exercise at 80 per cent of their maximum – most people who run popular marathons do not approach this, and so they should simply stick to their normal diets with moderate increases in carbohydrate.

Maintaining energy and hydration

During an event, for example, cycling or running, it is necessary to maintain energy and hydration. You shouldn't eat during the final two hours before the event and your last meal should have a high carbohydrate content. If the event is a long one, you can continue taking fluids right up to the start and you should then have 250 millilitres every 20 minutes during the event.

KEY POINTS

✓ Eat at least three good meals a day

✓ Balance your intake of different food types

✓ Fruit and vegetables are excellent sources of vitamins and other essential nutrients

✓ Avoid excess alcohol (28 units per week for a man and 21 for a woman)

Drug and lifestyle issues

DRUG USE

In the 1960s several cyclists died in amphetamine-related incidents, and the International Olympic Committee set up a special unit to eradicate drug use in sports. Testing for drugs was first introduced at the Olympic Games in Mexico in 1968, and steroid detection was first implemented during the Montreal Games in 1976.

Currently, the list of banned drugs includes stimulants, narcotics, anabolic steroids, beta-blockers, diuretics and peptide hormones. Drugs that remain under restriction include alcohol, marijuana, local anaesthetics and corticosteroids.

Officially, about two per cent of urine samples tested prove positive for drugs. This is thought to be an underestimate of the true prevalence, which may be as high as 20 per cent for the most popular drugs, amphetamines and steroids.

Certain drugs used for common ailments may actually be banned for competitive sport. For full details contact Sport England, 16 Upper Woburn Place, London WC1H 0QP (see page 95).

Anabolic steroids are drugs that increase muscle strength and lessen fatigue, and it is tempting to try them for competition. Apart from the risk of getting yourself banned, all drugs have potentially serious side effects and anabolic steroids are no different. In certain circumstances they can cause stunting of growth, changes in sexual function, breast development in men, acne and changes in the liver.

Full details of ergogenic aids and blood doping can be obtained from the Sports Council.

OTHER LIFESTYLE ISSUES

Coffee and tea

Some athletes believe that caffeine

drinks can stimulate the cardio-vascular system for a better result. Although there are theoretical benefits, no study has ever shown this to be true. Rather, the training effect of a lower heart rate is abolished by caffeine. Caffeine is also found in soft drinks such as cola and Lucozade. Most sports doctors advise moderation with caffeine.

Sleep

This is when your body repairs whatever damage it sustains during training, and recharges its energy stores, so it's vital to get enough while you're training if you are to do your best. On the other hand, if you are sleepless the night before a big race, resist the temptation to try artificial means of inducing sleep (such as pills and alcohol) as these will affect your performance the next day more than a sleepless night.

Smoking

Smoking has a significant effect on lung function and ventilation because it causes an increase in airway resistance. Immediately after smoking a cigarette this increased airway resistance can last for up to 80 minutes. Regular smoking also has other effects such as impairment of the lungs' capacity to absorb oxygen. This applies to passive smokers as well.

It is not easy to stop smoking but it can be done. You can get useful advice in the Health Education Council booklet – *Smokers' Guide to Non Smoking* – which should be available free from your health centre or doctor's surgery.

Minor illnesses

Everyone gets colds, with a runny nose or flu-like symptoms from time to time. When this happens, you need to reduce your training intensity or stop completely until you recover. Minor viral illnesses of this kind can cause inflammation of the membrane covering the heart which can trigger abnormal heart rhythms, especially during exercise. Sudden death in young people has occasionally been found to be caused by this condition. The viruses that produce minor respiratory symptoms may lead to inflammation of the heart muscle (myocarditis) or its lining (pericarditis).

Sex

There are many views as to whether you should abstain from sexual intercourse before physical activity. Some top athletes boast that they compete far better after intercourse and there are certainly no rules regarding this. Probably the most important thing is not to stay out very late at night before a competition the next day.

KEY POINTS

✓ Banned drugs include stimulants, narcotics, anabolic steroids, beta-blockers, diuretics and peptide hormones

✓ Certain medicines may be banned in competitive sport; check with your doctor

✓ Drink moderate amounts of caffeine, do not smoke, reduce or stop training if you have a cold or flu, and get adequate rest and social life

Sports injuries

HOW TO PREVENT INJURY

Contact team sports such as football, rugby and hockey have the highest rate of injury, followed by fencing, cricket and cycling. On average there are more than 30 injuries per 10,000 hours of play in football that require medical treatment on the field or attendance at an accident and emergency department. Combat sports such as boxing or judo have a lower rate of injury, but when accidents happen they may be devastating.

Injury prevention should be an essential part of every training programme. A first step towards this is a good understanding of how injuries occur in the first place. Recognising problems early and treating them skilfully increase the chance of a speedy recovery without complications. On occasions, it may even save lives.

The same processes of repair and healing take place in the body, almost irrespective of where the injury is. Different tissues heal at different rates, however, and some tissues heal less completely than others.

TECHNIQUE

Many injuries can be prevented or at least minimised with forethought and preparation. For starters, it is essential to learn the correct technique for your particular sport, because doing it the wrong way can cause harm. This applies especially when using gym equipment with complicated computerised settings – get an instructor to take you through the equipment and watch you while you use the machine. Often using the correct technique not only prevents injury but improves your performance.

FITNESS

Fitness also plays a role in preventing injury. Strong muscles 'hold' a joint tightly, whereas tired ones give way to sprains. However, the fitter an athlete is the more likely he or she is to push him- or herself, and the more susceptible he or she then becomes to injury. Finding the right balance can be difficult.

EQUIPMENT

The correct equipment for the sport is essential, both for optimum performance and to prevent accidents. Always wear adequate protection and support for vulnerable areas. Sports shops now carry a bewildering array of shoes for every possible activity. Although it is not necessary to buy the most advanced (and expensive) model, having the right shoe is important, so check that the one you're buying is suitable for what you do. Leave room for thick socks which are essential for extra cushioning, even on the warmest days.

More and more people are adopting a sensible attitude towards head protection. It is now normal for everyday cyclists to wear helmets. Helmets are also common for batsmen in cricket, despite the controversy and allegations of 'unmanliness' they provoked when players first started wearing them. Steeplechasers also wear helmets, and it has been reported that head protection worn during boxing training has reduced the frequency of knockouts from 4 per cent to 0.3 per cent of fights.

Face and eye protection are worn in sports such as hockey, squash and fencing. Gumshields protect the teeth, and the best ones are custom-made for the wearer by a dentist. Any protection worn by children and teenagers should be regularly refitted. Fencers wear a body suit, which in women includes breast protection, and groin protection is recommended for men in sports such as cricket and karate.

Very rarely, the protective gear itself causes problems. Motor-racing helmets sometimes do not allow for proper circulation of air, and the wearer may become light-headed or even pass out. Goggles cause eye damage if they are pulled partly off and rebound against the face. Ill-fitting equipment may also cause more damage than it is worth so do choose carefully.

RECOGNISE THE DANGERS AND PREVENT INJURY

Effective prevention of injury in sport and exercise depends on recognising the dangers in advance. There are three basic causes: trauma, overuse and environmental injury.

Trauma

This is a bodily injury, often found in contact and combat sports such as boxing, karate, football, rugby and

INJURY ACTION PLAN

It is inevitable that some time during exercise or sporting activity you'll either be injured yourself or witness an injury or accident. Follow these golden rules of injury management and prevention:

- Stay safe: in team sports play by the rules. Always exercise or train within your limitations. Ensure that you get fit for your sport or activity and make progress gradually.

- Stay cool: if you are injured don't panic. Stop the game, if necessary, or stop whatever activity you're doing. If someone else is injured, speak to him or her reassuringly and remain calm.

- Look and listen: if another person is injured, find out what happened, where the pain is, whether he or she can stand up or walk. Look for any obvious deformities. Compare sides when a limb is involved. DO NOT examine a lacerated eye in case you damage the eyeball itself.

- Touch: if you have an idea what has happened, gently use your hands to examine the injured part, comparing it with the other side of the body, head or limb.

- Get medical help: if you feel you need a professional opinion make sure you send for a doctor early rather than late.

- Remember – if someone has to go to hospital, do not give him or her anything to eat or drink in case a general anaesthetic is necessary.

hockey, and is usually caused by an opponent or by a piece of equipment such as a hockey stick.

Overuse

Overuse injuries are more common in aerobic activities which involve repeating a movement over a period of time. They are particularly common in racket sports, rowing and long-distance running, and tend to occur at specific sites such as the tendons around the ankle, knee, hip, shoulders and wrist. Looking after someone who has an injury of this kind may be more difficult as the person may try to carry on doing whatever caused it. This increases the risk of both recurrence and the development of a chronic (long-lasting) injury.

Environmental injury

This is caused by extremes of temperature, such as overheating while running on a hot day which can lead to dehydration, or hypothermia, which can be caused by immersion in water or the temperature conditions at high altitude and depth. Distance runners, climbers, skiers and participants in water sports are the high-risk groups.

WHERE TO GET HELP

If the injured person loses consciousness (no matter how briefly), they should be seen at an accident and emergency department (A&E). The same applies if they might have a broken or dislocated bone or if they need stitches or expert strapping.

If you've had a minor injury treated in A&E, you may have to see your own doctor for a follow-up examination or you may need to attend an outpatient clinic run by orthopaedic surgeons. A&E staff are trained to deal with common

BASIC RULES FOR PREVENTING INJURY

- Try to assess the particular risks of your activity or sport

- Know what your body is capable of and how fit you are; stay within your limitations

- Set realistic targets; try to make exercise and sport fun

- If you are playing games know the rules and stick to them

- Use the best equipment that you can afford or that which is recommended by experts

- Do not train through the pain of an injury; take expert or professional advice early rather than late

- Wear appropriate protective clothing or training gear

- Do not train when you have a cold or flu-like illness

- Try to train with a partner irrespective of whether you are training for a sport or for good health

- Make sure you warm up and cool down adequately

injuries, but will consult specialists for more major or unusual cases.

About 10 per cent of people who see their GPs do so for joint problems or sports injury. Many of these fall into the category of 'overuse', such as back strain, tennis elbow or knee problems. Your GP may prescribe suitable strapping, rest and pain relief, and may refer you to a specialist clinic if appropriate.

Many people treat simple injuries on their own. Chemists now stock a good range of joint supports, which can be used on mild sprains or strains, and pain-killers such as paracetamol and anti-inflammatories such as aspirin or ibuprofen may help. You can also buy skin preparations, in the form of creams, gels or sprays without a prescription. These work by 'irritating' the skin to produce warmth, which is soothing for muscle pain, or have a mild pain-killing action.

Any injury that causes significant swelling or does not improve within a few days should be seen by a doctor.

Some injuries respond well to injection with a local anaesthetic and steroid preparation. Local anaesthetic acts to relieve the pain for a few hours and the long-acting steroid preparation reduces the irritation around the injury. This type of therapy is particularly appropriate for chronic injuries where there is point tenderness, that is, when you can point to the area that is particularly troublesome. Typical examples include tennis elbow and golfer's elbow. One or two injections are enough to relieve the pain in most instances. The general rule of thumb is that no more than three injections of local anaesthetic and steroid should be given at the same site, because the risk of damage to tendons or ligaments (that is, rupture, tearing) increases with more frequent infections, as a result of a direct effect of steroids on these tissues. This type of injection should always be done by a doctor, preferably someone who has a specific interest in soft tissue/sports injuries.

There are a growing number of sport injury clinics within the National Health Service as well as within the private sector, and details of these can be obtained from your local hospital. Information on professionals within sports medicine, science and physio-therapy can be obtained from the National Sports Medicine Institute of the United Kingdom via the Sports Medicine Register (see page 95), which details their qualifications and publications, their practical involvement in sport, their profes-sional standing (which means at least three years' involvement in sports medicine as a major component of their work) and their membership of various of the professional sports medicine and science bodies. These may include the British Association of Sport and Medicine (BASM), the British Association of Sport and Exercise Sciences (BASES), the Association of Chartered Physiotherapists in Sports Medicine (ACPSM), Sports Nutrition Foundation (SNF), British Orthopaedic Sports Trauma Association (BOSTA) and the British Association of Trauma in Sports (BATS).

PHYSIOTHERAPY

Physiotherapy ranges from treatments to reduce pain and stiffness, to helping an injured athlete regain strength and flexibility. Active limbs do not take well to enforced rest, and specific exercises and procedures prescribed by the physiotherapist can shorten your recovery period.

Physiotherapists are normally attached to health centres and hospitals, and referrals may be made by your GP or hospital specialist although an increasing number of NHS and private physiotherapy-led clinics are now open access – you just phone for an appointment. You may be sent to see a physiotherapist if you need help in rehabilitation after a period of extended rest or immobilisation, for example, in a plaster cast.

'Physios' also use a variety of treatments to relieve pain and to restore your ability to move normally as soon as possible. They may use heat, supplied by hot baths, gel packs, lamps or diathermy, to provide relaxation, reduce muscle spasm and ease pain. Ultrasound may promote healing of soft tissue injuries and reduce swelling. Massage may also reduce spasm and swelling.

KEY POINTS

✓ Recognise the risks of your activity and take steps to prevent injury

✓ Use protective equipment: cycle helmets, gumshields, appropriate clothing and footwear

✓ Set realistic targets, play to the rules of the game and try to train with a partner

Different types of injury

THE BASIC PRINCIPLES

Sports injuries tend to be divided into two categories:

- soft tissue injuries (anything except bone)

- bony injury, which means either the bone is broken (fracture) or the bones are out of their normal alignment (dislocation).

To understand how bone and soft tissue (which includes skin, muscle, tendon, cartilage and ligaments) can become involved in injury, you need to understand how these structures are related to one another anatomically. The easiest way to do this is to study a typical joint, which is where many sports injuries strike. Joints are vulnerable because, although they are flexible to allow movement, they are also liable to twists and sprains.

In many activities they take the brunt of the weight (for instance, the knees in skiing) and/or repetitive movement.

Every joint is different, but the general principles of how bone, cartilage, tendon and so on are related to one another remain the same.

Joints are where two bones meet. The ends of the bones that move against each other are protected by cartilage. The joint is enclosed within a joint capsule (made up of fibrous tissue) which, on the innermost surface, is lined by a membrane called the synovial membrane. This produces a viscous fluid (the synovial fluid) which lubricates the bone surfaces within the capsule.

Muscles are attached to bones by tendons. Ligaments are supporting bands which connect one bone to the other, helping to hold the joint stable. Some joints have small thin bags called bursae

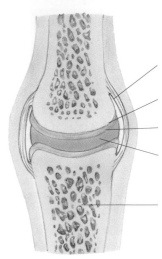

Many sports injuries involve joints. Joints allow the skeleton to move, but in so doing they are vulnerable to twists and sprains.

Ligaments – connect one bone to another

Cartilage – protects the ends of the bones

Synovial membrane – produces the lubricant synovial fluid

Synovial fluid – lubricates the joint capsule

Bone – hard framework that supports and protects soft tissues

(singular bursa), which add to the protection of the joint.

Actual joints are even more complex than this. For example, the knee joint is really a combination of three separate joints, and contains specially evolved tendons, ligaments and cartilage. Like any synovial joint, the ends of the knee bones are covered in white, smooth, articular cartilage. Second, the knee is unusual in having a pair of meniscus pads of shock-absorbing cartilage between the bones. It is these cartilages that get torn and sometimes need repair or replacement. A joint must be a complex structure to perform the wide range of movements demanded of it, but this also means that there is a lot of potential for things to go wrong.

SOFT TISSUE INJURIES

Skin

Skin may be cut or burned (by friction or by the sun). Bear in mind that cuts and scratches sustained on the sports field are likely to become infected, so you should always wash them thoroughly before applying any dressing. Make sure that your tetanus immunisation is always up to date. There is a layer of fat under the skin and, if the blood vessels in this are damaged, blood leaks into the tissues and creates the characteristic purple colour of a bruise.

Swelling and pain are natural defence mechanisms by which the body immobilises the injured part. Tissue damage is usually accom-

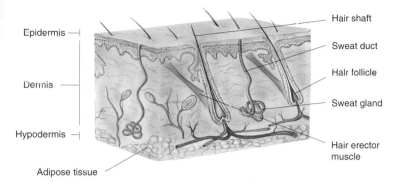

Epidermis ⊣

Dermis ⊣

Hypodermis ⊣

Adipose tissue

Hair shaft

Sweat duct

Hair follicle

Sweat gland

Hair erector muscle

The skin is your largest organ, weighing about four kilograms and covering about two square metres.

panied by some bleeding and the injury often triggers the production of tissue fluid, resulting in a swelling. The damage and swollen tissue stimulate nerve endings in the area, causing pain. In addition the swelling makes the injured part feel stiff, preventing you from using it. This allows repair processes to begin work and stops you from inflicting any further damage.

The bleeding and tissue fluid make the area feel warm and reddened – in other words, it becomes inflamed. The main aim of treatment for soft tissue injury is to reduce this inflammation and so speed up your recovery (see page 65).

Muscles

Injuries to muscles produce symptoms ranging from a 'minor twinge' when you move, which settles with time, to severe pain and fear brought on every time you do a particular exercise or movement. A pull or strain means that a few muscle fibres have been torn. A tear or rupture is more severe and is usually caused by a direct blow, such as a kick on the thigh. There may be bleeding, swelling and possibly a 'dead leg' caused by pressure on nerves. If you have severe symptoms of this kind, you should see a doctor on the day of the injury.

Putting an ice pack over the injured part will help relieve pain and swelling initially, then you need to apply a bandage and go to your local accident and emergency department if necessary.

Infection after muscle injury is very uncommon but sometimes cysts form inside the muscle if the bleeding has not settled adequately.

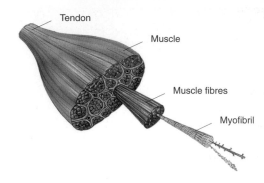

Muscle power – for movement and maintenance of posture.

These require medical treatment. A more common problem is shortening of the muscle as a result of formation of fibrous tissue which is less elastic than the muscle fibres themselves. This is why rehabilitation after any muscle injury must include stretching exercises to restore length and flexibility.

Thigh muscle injuries must be treated with particular respect or you may end up needing prolonged rest or surgical treatment. It's not a good idea to massage a thigh muscle injury because, in some cases, this will increase the size of the blood clot within it. This may become hardened and calcified or even form a lump of abnormal bone.

Tendons, ligaments, cartilage and bursae

Tendons can become inflamed with overuse: a condition known as tendonitis. The tendon becomes swollen, red and tender to the touch and hurts when you move it. You're most at risk of developing tendonitis if you perform one activity or movement regularly and intensely: runners get it in the Achilles' tendon and racket players in the wrist, for example. As well as rest, treatment usually includes some method of changing the way the tendon moves: for example, wearing a heel pad in Achilles' tendonitis. Treatment with non-steroidal analgesic drugs can also be helpful while the pain is severe and, if the problem does not clear up, you may need to have an injection of local anaesthetic and hydrocortisone into the covering of the tendon or possibly an operation to decompress the tendon.

Tendons can also be partially or completely torn. In a partial tear there is significant pain and discomfort and if the tear is complete you may be able to feel a

TREATING SOFT TISSUE INJURIES: 'RICE' PRINCIPLE

R = Relative rest

Some injuries may need complete rest because they are so serious but very often you will need only to limit your activities, cut back on training or change to another type of exercise. This is what is meant by relative rest and it allows you to maintain physical fitness while the injury heals.

I = Ice applied to the injured part

Ice reduces the amount of bleeding and bruising by cooling the blood vessels under the skin, making them constrict. It also has an anaesthetic effect, so it can relieve pain. When applying ice you must be careful not to burn the skin by direct application for too long. Either wrap the ice in a flannel or use a proper ice pack. Ice is an important component of treatment of an acute injury, but don't use an ice pack for longer than a period of 24 to 48 hours, during which you should apply it intermittently until the initial swelling goes down. Once the worst symptoms have subsided, usually after a week or so, there are many useful over-the-counter heat treatments for warming up the affected area. They are also worth using as part of your pre-match warm-up if you have a recurring injury.

C = Compressive bandaging

This is particularly effective in a limb injury. After you've applied an ice pack to the affected area several times for periods of 10 to 30 minutes, bandage it firmly if you can. This will also help to prevent further bleeding and swelling.

E = Elevation

Elevating the injured part allows the tissue fluid to drain away and will also help to reduce the size of the swelling and therefore relieve pain.

---

gap in the tendon.

Ligaments can be stretched, leading to partial or complete tears.

The word sprain is usually applied to minor tears of ligaments. These injuries result from twisting or wrenching of the affected joints. A complete tear will cause excessive pain, swelling, bruising or abnormal movement of the joint.

Bursae may become inflamed if they are constantly put under pressure and cartilage may be torn in more serious joint injuries. The knee joint contains the medial meniscus and the lateral meniscus – specially shaped cartilage at the top end of the tibia (the larger leg bone) – which can be torn by a fast, twisting action of the knee. This is a common football injury.

Always see a doctor for anything other than a minor injury, but first aid should follow what's called the RICE principle (see page 65)

BONY INJURIES

Fractured bones and dislocated joints are potentially serious, and should be treated by a doctor in the accident and emergency department. Bony injury often causes much soft tissue injury, bleeding into muscle, swelling and pain. You may feel faint or pass out with shock, pain or blood loss.

In some fractures the skin is broken by the jagged ends of the broken bones, although sometimes all you can actually see is a puncture wound on the skin. When this happens, infection may get into the bone, so this must always be regarded as a particularly serious injury.

Joints may simply be dislocated, or be fractured and dislocated. A dislocated joint is usually very painful, looks odd and the limb affected hangs loosely because you can't move it normally. All dislocations need urgent attention in accident and emergency because, the sooner they are put back, the better the outcome.

First aid for bony injuries

If the person is in considerable pain the quickest way to relieve it is to splint the injury. This may involve the use of a simple first aid splint or splinting an injured leg to the uninjured one or a damaged finger to its neighbour (buddy strapping). Injured arms can be made more comfortable with a sling or bandage. In such situations ask the person what feels most comfortable and try to immobilise the limb in that position. Do not let the person eat or drink in case he or she needs an anaesthetic later.

Once in accident and emergency, an X-ray will be taken of the injury. Some fractures can be 'reduced' (realigned) using local anaesthetic techniques and sedation without an operation. Other fractures require 'internal fixation' – that is, they need metal plates and screws to hold the bones in place while healing takes place. An operation is required. A general anaesthetic cannot be given until FOUR hours

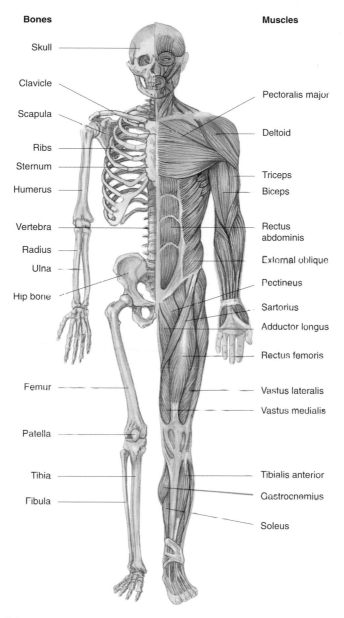

Bones

Skull

Clavicle

Scapula

Ribs

Sternum

Humerus

Vertebra

Radius

Ulna

Hip bone

Femur

Patella

Tibia

Fibula

Muscles

Pectoralis major

Deltoid

Triceps

Biceps

Rectus abdominis

External oblique

Pectineus

Sartorius

Adductor longus

Rectus femoris

Vastus lateralis

Vastus medialis

Tibialis anterior

Gastrocnemius

Soleus

The skeleton protects and provides support for the soft tissues of the body. The joints connect bones and allow movement.

after the last drink, and SIX hours after the last meal, because vomiting and choking under an anaesthetic are dangerous.

Most reduced fractures are held with a plaster cast, to immobilise the limb. Expect to wear the cast for about six weeks, but the precise timing varies from one person to another.

SKIN INJURIES AND PROBLEMS

Blisters
These are caused by shearing forces, such as the movement of the foot inside a training shoe, which is one reason why you should always wear well-fitting shoes and thick socks. When possible, smearing the skin with petroleum jelly may prevent friction. If you do get a blister, puncture it with a sterile needle, then cover it with a dressing to prevent further damage.

Abrasions
Wash broken and grazed skin with soap and water or an antiseptic agent to remove dirt, then cover it with a sterile dressing.

Cuts and lacerations
A cut is an injury produced by a sharp edge such as broken glass or the blade of a knife, whereas a laceration is a ragged cut usually caused by a blunt object. Cover the injury with a sterile dressing and apply pressure to stop bleeding. If the cut or laceration is minor you can wash it with soap and water, but more serious cuts or lacerations and those that may contain foreign bodies or that fail to stop bleeding need to be seen by a doctor. (See page 65 for control of serious bleeding.)

Bruises
These are caused by bleeding under the skin; very extensive bruises are called haematomas. A haematoma is a collection of blood within a space, for example, in the quadriceps muscle on the thigh or in the soft tissue around the eye (black eye), or under the skin of the shin bone. Haematomas can also occur within joints and in the chest, abdominal or skull cavities. Minor bruises require little treatment other than cooling. Haematomas may require medical attention and it's wise to go to the hospital accident and emergency department. Haematomas usually occur in the large muscle groups, particularly quadriceps muscle of the thigh. Sometimes a haematoma can be very large indeed and it may be necessary to accelerate healing by aspirating it under aseptic conditions. This usually involves having a local anaesthetic so that a large-bore needle can be inserted to draw out the blood into a syringe.

Burns

Other than in motor sport, burns are usually caused by friction rather than physical heat. Wrestlers and judo practitioners may get mat burns (grazes) while grass burns are associated with playing on synthetic turf. Burns may also be caused by one body part rubbing repeatedly against another (such as inner thighs in runners) or clothing (nipple burn in women runners). Covering the area with petroleum jelly can prevent this.

Other burns should be immediately cooled with tap water or an ice pack and usually no other treatment will be necessary.

Fungal infections

The moist environment created when you sweat for long periods encourages fungal infections such as 'athlete's foot' or 'jock itch'. Communal showers and swimming pools are often breeding grounds for the organisms leading to these infections. Personal hygiene is also important to discourage infection.

Fungal infections cause an irritating itch between the toes or in the groin crease. You pick them up through direct contact with floors, shower rooms and other moist surfaces which actually harbour the infection. Using the same towel all week or sharing towels with other people may be a factor too.

If possible you should have two or even three sets of training gear so that one is always freshly washed. If you are using only one set of training clothes wash them as regularly as possible, at least twice a week, and leave them to dry overnight. If you're involved with managing children and teenagers, try to arrange for training clothes or team clothes to be laundered on a regular basis, so that they are fresh at least once a week. The importance of fresh kit cannot be over-emphasised.

To prevent athlete's foot, make a point of washing your feet quickly in warm water, without soaking them, at least once a day and certainly after every training session. Dry them gently and wait several minutes before putting on your socks which should also be changed daily. By all means use talcum powder if you want to once your feet are dry but remember that it is no substitute for proper drying, especially between the toes. Nylon socks actually increase sweating so opt for wool or cotton with a minimum of synthetic fibres.

You can buy antifungal preparations to treat athlete's foot or groin from the chemist without a prescription. If there is no improvement after two weeks consult your doctor. Spread a towel to stand on after showering to avoid passing on the infection to other people, and don't use the towel for anything else.

Do not walk with bare feet on surfaces used by others. Use a separate towel to dry the groin creases and keep your underwear clean and fresh.

Verrucas and corns

You are vulnerable to getting footwarts (verrucas) if you take part in activities with bare feet such as swimming, karate or judo. A verruca always occurs in the sole of the foot and feels as though you are walking on a small pebble. Specialist treatment from either a doctor or chiropodist is required.

A corn is a thickening of normal skin resulting from friction from shoes, usually at the pressure points. Treat it with lanolin and then abrade it with an emery board (a cardboard nail file).

FACIAL INJURIES

Our psychological and social well-being depends very much on how we look and having a heavily scarred face can be stigmatising. You need to protect important areas such as your eyes, ears, nose and mouth from any injury.

Cauliflower ear

This is common in combat sports such as boxing and wrestling and in contact sports such as rugby. It results from a blow to the area which causes bleeding under the skin of the ear. Apply an ice pack for first aid, but all such injuries should be seen as soon as possible by the club doctor, who will remove the haematoma and prevent its recurrence by applying pressure dressing or prescribing appropriate medication.

Broken nose

This often follows a hard blow and can occur with or without deformity of the nose. Usually, when nasal cartilages dislocate from the bone they cause deformity, although in some cases the bone itself actually breaks. If there is a break in the skin or obvious deformity, you need to get to hospital as soon as possible. The nose can often be pushed back into position under local anaesthetic, and will look normal afterwards. In sports where a broken nose is a recurrent problem, these injuries produce the classic picture of the 'boxer's nose'.

Broken cheekbone

You can feel this bone just in front of your ear and where it passes across your face to your nose. It gives the middle part of your face its fullness. When it's broken, your face on that side may look flattened and there may be blood in the white of the eye. You may find it difficult to open your mouth so you have to talk through your teeth. An operation is necessary to correct the deformity so you must go to accident and emergency.

Fractures of the jaw

The symptoms include pain in the jaw and you may have trouble talking or gritting your teeth and notice blood in your saliva. You need to get to hospital straightaway as all fractures of the jaw need medical attention. The jaw may have to be 'wired' – that is, fixed in position with the mouth closed – to allow healing. Remember to wear a gumshield in contact and combat sports because this prevents many injuries.

Dental injuries

These are almost 100 per cent preventable simply by wearing a properly custom-built gumshield for any high-risk sports. Make sure that children's gumshields are renewed regularly as they grow. Ask your dentist about this service.

If the tooth is still attached to the gum, try to return it to its original position by gentle pressure. If it has been completely dislodged wash it and try to push it back into its socket. If this is not possible, put it inside its owner's mouth between the gum and lip. Once this has been done, the person should go straight to a dentist. If a tooth is replaced within the hour it may be saved.

DO NOT PLACE LOOSE TEETH INTO THE MOUTH OF ANYONE WHO IS NOT FULLY CONSCIOUS.

Eye injuries

Eye injuries are very common, and almost 90 per cent of them are preventable. About one-third are serious enough to require hospital admission for treatment. Unfortunately such injuries predominantly affect young men under 25, including a very large number of children, half of whom will suffer permanent loss of their field of vision or of the ability to focus properly.

High-risk activities include any sport involving missiles (balls, shuttlecocks) or rackets or sticks, combat sports such as karate, boxing and contact sports such as football and rugby.

The most common serious injury is caused by a direct blow to the eye by a fist or a ball. This compresses the eyeball into its socket and leads to potentially serious complications throughout the eye, including rupture of the eyeball. The most visible sign is a black eye, caused by bruising, but this in itself is not harmful. It may, however, make examination of the eye more difficult. Otherwise, the cornea may be scratched, the iris torn or the lens dislocated.

If you are in intense pain and feel unwell and sick, this is a sign that the pressure within the eye is increasing (as a result of bleeding) and urgent medical help is needed.

Other mishaps include torn eyelids, scratched corneas, grit or dust in the eye. Wearing goggles prevents the cornea becoming inflamed from contact with chlorine in the swimming pool, and the right protection can prevent your eyes becoming raw after too much exposure to ultraviolet radiation, as in snow-blindness in skiers and mountaineers.

All eye injuries should be quickly assessed on the spot. If there is any pain, swelling, change in vision or change in the shape of the pupil, get medical attention urgently. Simple problems like corneal scratches and grit in the eye can be dealt with by the A&E staff; more serious problems will receive the attention of the eye surgeon.

SHOULDER, ARM AND HAND INJURIES

Dislocated shoulder

This is caused by a fall on to the outstretched hand. The shoulder looks deformed, square in appearance, and the arm appears too long. The injured person supports the arm with his other hand. Diagnosis is confirmed by X-ray, which will also reveal any fractures near the dislocation.

Treatment:

● Reduction of the dislocation (putting it back) should take place in hospital. This can be done under sedation, but often a general anaesthetic is needed.

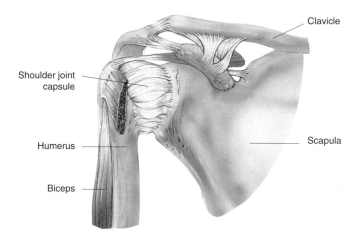

Rotator cuff lesions: this is the medical term often used to describe a group of soft tissue problems around the joint capsule of the shoulder.

- Healing of the soft tissues may take 2–4 weeks. After this the shoulder may be exercised, but return to full sport, especially contact sports, should be delayed for 2–3 months.

- In some cases, actual shoulder dislocation, or the feeling that the joint may dislocate, may become a recurrent problem. This can have serious consequences for the patient's sporting prospects, and needs to be assessed by an orthopaedic surgeon. The joint may be repaired under general anaesthetic.

Broken collar bone

This is caused by a fall on the outstretched hand and is especially common in young people and children. There is usually obvious deformity and the skin may be broken. The injured person supports the damaged arm with his other hand.

Treatment:

- This injury is managed in hospital, usually with the application of a sling or braces.

Acromioclavicular joint damage

There is a small joint between the collar bone and the shoulder blade, at the tip of the shoulder. It can be damaged during contact sports, as a result of a fall on to the point of the shoulder or the outstretched arm. There is tenderness and swelling over the affected area and sometimes a step can be seen between the end of the collar bone and the shoulder itself.

Treatment:

- The injury should be examined in the accident and emergency department. Usually, the arm is placed in a broad sling.

- Once the pain subsides, the arm and shoulder can be exercised with pendular movements.

- In more serious cases, the joint may need repair with screws, which are removed after six weeks.

Rotator cuff lesions

This is the medical term to describe a group of soft tissue problems around the joint capsule of the shoulder. Sports that require repetitive overarm movement – such as bowling a cricket ball, swimming, serving a tennis ball – can lead to irritation and inflammation of the tendons and bursa around the shoulder. Overarm movements become painful, which can badly affect sporting performance. Acute shoulder tendonitis causes rapid-onset pain on lifting the arm away from the body. Rotating the arm may also be painful. Chronic shoulder tendonitis tends to affect weekend sportsmen. The pain develops gradually over several weeks. The shoulder may not be tender, but it is still painful to make an arc with the arm.

Treatment:

- In mild cases, resting the arm in a broad sling for a few days, plus regular anti-inflammatory medication, should suffice.

- In more severe cases, injections of local anaesthetic mixed with steroids into the shoulder joint may be helpful.

- GPs may treat mild cases, but more severe cases are referred to hospital specialists.

Tennis elbow

Pain on the outer part of the elbow, especially when you're gripping a racket, is called tennis elbow and the area over your outer elbow may also feel tender. This is an overuse injury common in racket sports but can be caused by any repetitive movement.

Treatment:

- Apply ice packs and take several days' rest. Avoid moving your arm in such a way that it hurts.

- Use a supportive bandage or

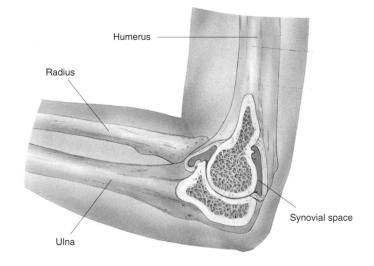

Cross-section through the elbow joint.

strapping for the muscles of the upper forearm.

- Take simple pain-killers or an anti-inflammatory medicine such as aspirin or ibuprofen

- Consider changing the size of your racket handle.

- If you are still in pain after a few days, see your doctor who may give you local anaesthetic and steroid injections.

Golfer's elbow

This affects the inside of the elbow and is caused by forceful stretching of the ligaments and muscles on that side. It is common in golfers and racket players.

Treatment: As for tennis elbow.

Wrist strain

This is caused by repetitive or unaccustomed use of the wrist and is common in racket sports. There is pain on the back of the wrist and thumb with a crunching sensation as the tendons move.

Treatment:

- Apply the RICE principle (see page 65).

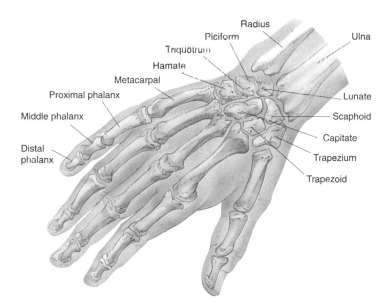

Radius
Pisiform
Triquetrum
Ulna
Hamate
Metacarpal
Proximal phalanx
Middle phalanx
Lunate
Distal phalanx
Scaphoid
Capitate
Trapezium
Trapezoid

The wrist and hand contain very many bones.

- Anti-inflammatory drugs are often helpful, provided you don't have any troublesome side effects.

- Splinting may ease the pain.

- Avoid repeating the movements that produce the symptoms.

- If you injure your wrist in a fall, always get it checked out by a doctor to rule out a hard-to-detect fracture of a small wrist bone called the scaphoid bone. If the scaphoid is fractured, there will be tenderness in the area between the wrist and base of the thumb, and pain when the thumb is pulled backwards. Scaphoid injuries are diagnosed by means of an X-ray, and your arm will be placed in a plaster cast for six to twelve weeks.

Finger and thumb injuries

Strains, fractures and dislocations are common; strains or tears to the ligaments at the base of the thumb are especially important. Such injuries cause severe pain.

Treatment:

- Thumb injuries should always be treated in hospital because you can't grip if you can't use your thumb, whereas finger sprains, while very painful, do not usually require medical advice.

- Fingers can get dislocated in contact sports such as rugby. If the skin is undamaged, the dislocation can be reduced at the time by pulling the finger straight, allowing the joint to slip back into position. Try this only once and if you fail take the person to hospital. If it works, strap the injured finger to the one next to it (buddy strapping) to relieve the pain.

- Finger fractures should also be seen in A&E. Often immobilisation by buddy strapping is all that is required; however, more severe fractures may need to be held in place with a wire, which is inserted under general anaesthetic.

LOWER LIMB INJURIES

Clicking hip

You may develop this if you do a lot of stretching exercises: as you stand with your legs apart and stretch you hear a loud clunk which isn't usually painful. A clicking hip is fairly common and is caused by a tight band of muscle or tendon sliding over the outer part of the hip joint. If you do get pain with it, see your doctor.

Adductor muscle tears

The muscles on the inside of the thigh can be torn during over-

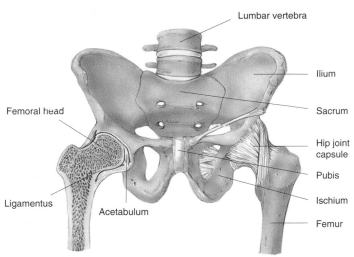

The hip joint is a ball and socket joint, the femoral head being held in the acetabulum by strong ligaments.

enthusiastic stretching exercises or when making a football tackle. Sometimes a splinter of bone is pulled off as the muscle tears. The injury is very painful, particularly on stretching or whenever the muscle is tensed.

Treatment:

- Apply the RICE principle as quickly as possible (see page 65).

- Once the initial pain has passed, make an effort to use the muscle gently in stretching movements but always within the limits of pain.

- Take soluble aspirin or ibuprofen at the time of the injury and four-

hourly afterwards for the first day to ease the pain.

Groin pain

This type of injury mostly affects people taking part in soccer, handball, ice hockey, skiing, athletics and horse riding. Groin pain can be the result of an overstretch injury or inflammation of tendons in the thigh and abdomen. The arrangement of muscles in this region is complex, and many muscles are vulnerable to overuse pain. Groin pain may also be caused by unstable pelvic bones.

You normally notice a gradual ache in the groin which becomes worse after activity. It may cause difficulties with kicking a ball or hurt when you cough or get out of bed, for example.

Treatment:

- Relative rest.

- Take an analgesic (pain-killer) such as soluble aspirin.

- Begin gentle remobilisation after several days.

- Physiotherapy exercises.

- If the problems persist, you may require surgery to repair a tear in the muscle of the lower abdominal wall or even a small early hernia.

Thigh injuries

The thigh muscles (the quadriceps at the front and the hamstrings at the back) may get bruised, usually following a direct blow which causes a sudden pain followed by a deep aching and sometimes obvious swelling.

Treatment:

- Use the RICE principle (see page 65) and, if necessary, spend a day or two in bed to let the swelling settle.

- Never massage a thigh injury because this may produce complications (including abnormal bone formation) and delay healing.

- Carefully limit all activities for the few days after injury to prevent complications.

- See a doctor in the accident and emergency department within 24 hours of the injury if you have a lot of swelling and severe pain.

Muscle strains and ruptures

A direct severe blow is the usual cause: you may experience the feeling of a 'dead leg', tenderness at the site of the injury and sometimes you may be able to feel a gap in the muscle. It hurts when you try to tense the muscle. Alternatively you may have overused one or more muscles in the thighs or abdomen, making it painful to move in certain ways.

Muscle strains causing pain in the pubic region (adductor longus muscle), the inner thigh (iliopsoas), the front of the thigh (quadriceps) and the upper or lower thigh (hamstrings) are all relatively common.

Treatment:

- Apply the RICE principle.

- Take simple analgesic drugs.

- Start gentle exercises once the pain has settled.

- If the symptoms haven't gone after two or three days see a doctor.

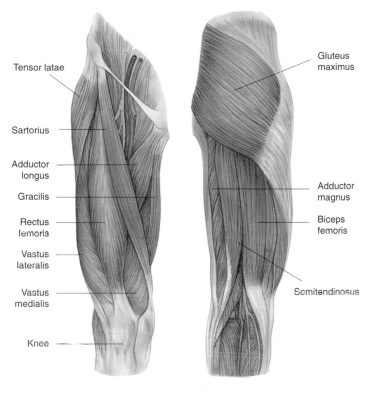

Tensor latae

Sartorius

Adductor longus

Gracilis

Rectus femoris

Vastus lateralis

Vastus medialis

Knee

Gluteus maximus

Adductor magnus

Biceps femoris

Semitendinosus

Front

Back

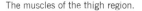

The muscles of the thigh region.

You may get repeated muscle strains because of the formation of scar tissue which is not as flexible as normal muscle. With all muscle injuries, adequate rest and gradual return to training are critical, because a quick return may cause recurrence.

Make sure you don't overtrain and, if your problem is severe, you may need to alter your activities, so that less strain is placed on the same muscle.

THE KNEE

Runner's knee

This is pain in the region of the knee cap caused when it repeatedly rubs against the lower end of the thigh bone. Looked at through an arthroscope (a small viewing device inserted under general anaesthetic), the knee-cap cartilage may be abnormal, but even if it is not you may still be in considerable pain. Women are more prone to this problem than men. The cause is thought to be a slight misplacement of the knee joint and quadriceps muscle, or a slight deformity in the way the leg moves, which comes to light only with training.

You may feel pain and clicking behind the knee cap after training and/or sitting for a long time. Going down stairs is also painful and you may see a small swelling.

Treatment:

- Apply the RICE principle.

- Strengthen the quadriceps muscle: sit upright with your knees bent at 90 degrees, then straighten the leg. A light weight may be strapped to the foot for more intense exercise.

- Consider a carefully balanced muscle retraining programme.

- Avoid sitting still with the knee bent for long periods; keep the knee mobile.

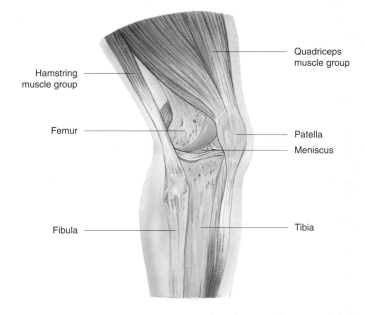

Hamstring muscle group

Femur

Fibula

Quadriceps muscle group

Patella

Meniscus

Tibia

Front three-quarter section of the knee joint.

- If none of this helps, you may need to see a specialist who will decide whether you need surgery. Arthroscopy is a telescopic examination of the knee joint during which therapeutic surgery can be performed; other forms of surgery involve exposing the knee cap and either making the under-surface smoother or realigning the knee cap so that it no longer rubs against the lower end of the thigh bone. The attraction of arthroscopy is that you can get back to your normal activities relatively quickly afterwards.

Knee ligament injuries

The knee has four main ligaments: two inside the joint (cruciate ligaments) and two on either side of the knee (collateral ligaments). Most injuries are the result of twisting movements (such as in a football tackle) or a direct blow. Minor sprains may cause tenderness in the inside or outside of the knee joint. In major injuries the knee will 'bend' the wrong way. Paradoxically, complete tears of ligaments are less painful than partial tears. Your knee may feel unstable when walking or running, especially when changing direction.

Treatment:

- Use the RICE regimen (see page 65) for first aid.

- Have the knee examined by a doctor if possible because you may need surgery to remove blood from the joint or to repair the ligaments if it's unstable.

- After surgery, the knee will be placed in a plaster cast for four to six weeks, then you will follow an exercise regimen involving increasingly rapid running movements.

Torn cartilage (meniscus injury)

The meniscus cartilages are two C-shaped wedges between the femoral (thigh bone) and tibial (shin bone) surfaces of the knee joint. They are attached to the tibia at its upper end and are thought to act as shock absorbers and to allow the even spreading of joint fluid. When torn they can become loose inside the joint and interfere with its movements.

Soccer alone accounts for almost 70 per cent of meniscus injuries. The knee suddenly gives way or locks and can't be immediately straightened.

Treatment:

- The RICE regimen should be your first recourse.

- If your knee locks, swells, is persistently painful or gives

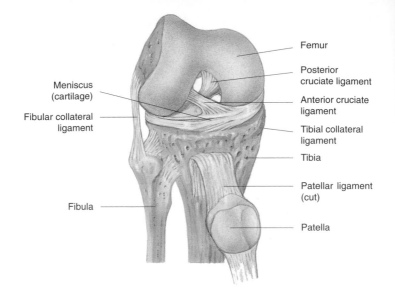

The three bones of the knee are held together by a network of strong ligaments.

way, you need a medical opinion. You will have an arthroscopy (see page 81) and the torn cartilage will either be repaired or, if the tear is too extensive, it may be partially or completely removed.

- No artificial cartilages are used in this country at present.

LOWER LEG INJURIES

The two bones of the lower leg are the tibia which bears the body weight and the fibula, the strut-like bone to which the three groups of lower leg muscles are attached. The two in the calf are the gastrocnemius and soleus, which form a tendon that is inserted into the heel bone, the Achilles' tendon. These muscles provide the propulsive force for actions such as sprinting and jumping.

At the front of the leg another group of muscles pulls the ankle upwards – you can feel them tense and relax as you move your foot up and down. Combined muscle action allows you to turn the foot outwards or inwards.

Stress fractures

These are overuse injuries. A stress fracture is a crack in the bone caused by repeatedly striking the foot on the ground and can occur in many sports including football and

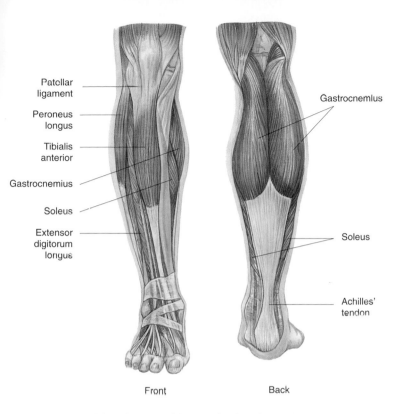

Principal muscles of the lower right leg – front and back.

long distance running. (They usually affect the lower limb but can also occur in the bones of the spine and even in the ribs in one golfer!) The classic symptom is pain provoked by activity and the area over the fracture will be tender.

A stress fracture can usually be diagnosed by an X-ray two or three weeks later when signs of bone healing become visible or at an earlier stage by means of a bone scan.

Treatment:

- If a fracture is in a weight-bearing bone then rest is essential; otherwise just reducing your level of activity for about six to eight weeks will usually allow it to heal.

- Allow at least a further four weeks before starting graduated training again and be prepared to slow the pace if exercise triggers any pain.

Shin splints

This condition is usually the result of repetitive movements which lead to inflammation of the tendons and muscle attached to the shin, but symptoms can also be the result of a stress fracture or swelling of the muscle. You feel pain down the front of the leg, usually in the lower half from the mid-point of the tibia bone down to the ankle. It gradually increases and eventually you feel pain both during and after running and even while walking.

Your calf may be tight and you may get cramps or occasionally numbness of the foot. Novices training on hard roads or who are in poor physical condition are particularly susceptible.

Treatment:

- Apply the RICE principle (see page 65).

- Reduce your training programme so that it isn't painful.

- Always exercise on a soft surface like grass.

- Wear good quality absorbent footwear.

- If you suspect your running style may be faulty, get advice from an experienced coach.

- If all these measures fail seek medical advice.

Tibial compartment syndrome

This is a form of shin splint that affects the muscles on the front of the lower leg. They lie between two bones, the tibia and fibula, and they are strongly encased in a tough fibrous tissue called fascia.

Sometimes after strenuous activity or even a direct injury this part of your leg swells, compressing the artery which is its blood supply. Symptoms are severe pain on the front of your leg and sometimes you may feel a numbness between the first and second toes.

Treatment:

- Stop your exercise.

- Elevate the limb and apply the RICE regimen.

- See your doctor because you may need surgery to decompress the leg.

- The condition can also occur in untrained people in a more chronic form. This doesn't need urgent treatment and usually changing your training programme so as to stop the pain works well but, if not, you may need surgery.

Achilles' tendon

The Achilles' tendon is a potential weak spot in top-class athletes who do a lot of road running, and middle-aged and older exercisers. The most common problems are rupture and tendonitis.

• **Achilles' tendon rupture:** Older exercisers (middle age onwards) are most vulnerable, but this problem can affect young people, especially after a blow to the tendon. The tendon becomes very painful and it may be difficult to stand. Gentle examination will reveal a gap which can be felt in the tendon.

Treatment:

• This must be carried out in hospital. Surgery is one option and, if it is necessary, it must be performed as soon as possible. You will have a plaster cast on your leg for about six weeks afterwards.

• An alternative is simply to put the leg in a cast for a longer period (eight weeks) followed by a longer programme of rehabilitation.

• While the injury is healing, you'll have to walk with your heel raised to relax the tendon, and you'll be given exercises to stretch and strengthen your calf muscles.

• Whichever form of treatment you are given, the outcome will be much the same after six to twelve months. The tendon will be as strong as before and you should be able to use your leg normally. One man retained a world karate championship title despite sustaining a traumatic rupture of the Achilles' tendon during training.

• **Tendonitis:** This is inflammation of the covering of the Achilles' tendon. It usually starts with a vague ache which gets progressively worse until the whole tendon becomes swollen and very tender to touch; you may also feel crackling as your foot moves up and down.

Treatment:

• Rest is essential after you've applied the RICE regimen.

• Wearing a heel raise of one to two centimetres inside your shoe can relieve symptoms.

• You may require physiotherapy.

• Anti-inflammatory drugs can help.

• In chronic cases surgical treatment is necessary.

• When the symptoms are subsiding, you should avoid

stressing the tendon. Run or walk on grass rather than hard surfaces when possible, avoiding hills, and continue to wear the heel raise.

Calf strain

This can be caused by overuse or a direct blow although there may be no obvious cause in an older person. Your calf will be painful and swollen and you may be able to feel a gap in the muscle.

Treatment:

- Apply the RICE principle at once and continue with it for 48 hours.

- Begin gentle stretching exercises within the limits of pain after 48 hours.

- Consult your doctor if you can feel a gap in the muscle

Cramp

This mostly affects the legs but you can get it in any group of muscles. It is a painful and persistent spasm of a muscle caused by over-contraction of a muscle or a group of muscles, sometimes because you are dehydrated or cold. Although the exact cause of cramp isn't fully understood, it may be related to the accumulation of waste products within the muscle. As well as being very painful, the muscle is tightly contracted.

Treatment:

- Stop whatever activity you were doing.

- If the cramp is in your calf, gently stretch the muscle by pushing the sole of the foot upwards while straightening the leg. This often allows the muscle to relax.

- Once the cramped muscle is released, you need to rest.

FOOT PROBLEMS AND INJURIES

Blisters

Blisters are caused by shearing forces often associated with poor footwear or wrinkled socks.

Treatment:

- Prick the blister with a sterile needle.

- Drain the fluid.

- Cover the blister with tape or a dressing to protect it and enable you to carry on exercising.

Jogger's toe

This is common in people who do long-distance running and can be very painful. It appears as a bruise under the toenail and is caused by ill-fitting training shoes.

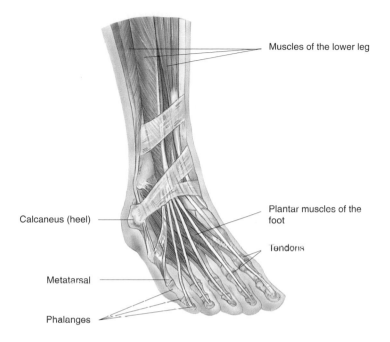

Muscles of the lower leg

Plantar muscles of the foot

Tendons

Calcaneus (heel)

Metatarsal

Phalanges

Sports injuries frequently occur in the foot and ankle.

Treatment:

- See your doctor, who will probably pierce the nail and drain the blood.

Heel spur syndrome (plantar fasciitis, policeman's heel)

Your heel and the arch of your foot will be painful and may be extremely tender to touch. An X-ray will reveal the heel spur, which is often associated with a strained arch or the so-called policemen's heel. Whether the spur itself is significant remains controversial. The cause of plantar fasciitis is poor instep support and repetitive activities (such as walking the beat). These are both related to unsuitable or inadequate footwear.

Treatment: When the pain is severe:

- Apply the RICE principle over 48 hours.

- Work out what is causing the problem so you can eliminate whatever it is.

- Wear a heel pad in your shoe.

- Do stretching exercises to stretch the calf muscles and the Achilles' tendon.

- If there is no improvement, see a doctor. Injecting the heel with local anaesthetic and steroid can cure the condition.

KEY POINTS

✓ Injuries may be to the soft tissues (skin, muscles, tendons, nerves, ligaments) or to bone

✓ Apply the RICE principle when treating soft tissue injuries

✓ Cuts, lacerations, burns, infections and suspected broken bones may require medical treatment

✓ Eye and teeth injuries may be prevented in almost 90 to 100 per cent of cases

Serious injuries and emergencies

An emergency might involve unconsciousness, the suspicion of a neck injury, a broken bone, persistent bleeding, chest pain or even cardiac arrest. You will be able to deal with these situations if you have acquired the necessary skills on a basic first aid course (see Useful addresses on page 94).

Practice under expert guidance is the key to confidence in dealing effectively with emergencies. If you do have to do so, it is essential that you or someone else controls any spectators who may hamper attempts at treatment by giving all kinds of advice.

If you really know what to do, you will not have to listen to them.

HEAD INJURIES

Any bump on the head that is associated with loss of memory or loss of consciousness should be regarded as potentially serious. Other warning signs include nausea and vomiting or drowsiness. If in doubt, the victim should be taken to the accident and emergency department.

Why head injuries are different

Unlike many other sports injuries, they can be life-threatening, usually as a result of the development of secondary complications rather than the severity of the initial impact. Complications include bleeding inside the brain, brain swelling and infection.

Many of the problems associated with these complications are preventable and people involved in sport should know what to do. In contact or combat sports such as football, rugby or boxing, someone who suffers a head injury that affects their level of consciousness is likely to sustain another – possibly even more serious – injury.

Concussion

This is a knockout or a period of loss of memory after a bump on the head (known as post-traumatic amnesia – PTA). In a knockout there is sudden loss of consciousness which may last a few minutes or hours. Alternatively, after a bump on the head the person may have no immediate recall of what has happened even though he or she may appear to be talking normally. In such instances you need to ask some specific questions (see below).

Concussion is dangerous because, even in a minor injury that is associated with loss of consciousness or memory, complications can set in.

The person may be knocked out for several seconds or minutes, then appear to recover completely, but may also sustain loss of memory (post-traumatic amnesia) for events after the injury.

Treatment:

- Even if the person seems to have made a full recovery after a minute or two, they may be functioning automatically without really being aware of what is happening.

- To avoid the risk of a second injury (especially if you're playing a contact sport) get the injured player to sit on the sidelines for a while.

- Take your time to assess the person and if there is any doubt obtain medical advice. Ask:

    1 Do you know where you are and what happened?

    2 Do you know who you are?

    3 What's your address?

    4 What's your job?

    5 Do you have a headache or feel sick?

- Then check whether they are moving in a coordinated way – can they hop and touch their nose with their index finger? Can they obey simple commands? Do their eyes follow your fingers as you move them and are their pupils of equal size?

Unconsciousness

Treatment:

- Unless you suspect a neck injury, an unconscious and breathing person should be placed carefully in the coma position

- Check that the airway is clear and that the person is breathing

- Check their pulse

- Cover any wounds and keep them warm

- GET MEDICAL HELP IMMEDIATELY.

Neck injury

This is potentially very serious. There may be damage to the spinal cord which can lead to paralysis or death. High-risk sports are diving, rugby, gymnastics, American football, motor racing, winter sports and horse riding.

Possible causes include head-on tackles, collapsed scrums, dives into a shallow pool, falling off a horse or a rock, falling badly on to a trampoline.

Symptoms and signs

- Numbness or tingling of the arms or legs

- Paralysis – check whether the person can move his or her arms or legs.

Treatment:

- Stay cool

- Look and listen

- Do not attempt to move the person without expert help.

LESS SERIOUS INJURIES

Acute cervical sprain

This is an injury that occurs frequently in contact and high-velocity activities including motor sport and parachuting. After a twisting movement, the person may develop pain in the neck and be unable to move it normally. They may also feel pain or even tingling in their arms. Although they should go to hospital for an X-ray, no damage may show up because this type of injury is often a result of stretching the supporting ligaments or joints. A person who repeatedly suffers this type of injury – from heading a football, for example – may eventually develop neck changes visible on X-ray.

Treatment:

- Anti-inflammatory drugs are usually given for seven days or until neck movements return.

- Persistent pain will require further investigation and possibly physiotherapy and neck traction.

CHEST INJURY

This may be caused by direct blows, muscle strains, broken ribs, punctured lung or a heart attack. Possible symptoms include persistent pain in the chest, or pain on breathing, sneezing or laughing;

a heart attack is a possible cause of sweating, coldness, clamminess, shivering, nausea and vomiting.

Minor chest injuries

For direct blows, muscle strains, broken ribs and bruised cartilages, you should first apply an ice pack to the injury, then sit the person down and arrange to have them checked by a doctor.

A punch or a blow to the midriff will lead to difficulty in breathing, usually for about 30 to 60 seconds. Don't move or touch the injured person, except to loosen any tight clothing. Do not apply pressure of any sort to the injured area in case there is internal damage. If the player is slow to recover, or is in continued difficulties, get urgent medical help.

THE FIRST AID KIT

Make sure that you buy a well-equipped first aid bag suitable for your sport. It should contain at least the following:

- Dressings including sticking plasters, crêpe bandages, sterile wound pads, adhesive strapping, eye pads

- Pen torch

- Antiseptic cream or lotion, povidone–iodine solution or spray (or some other antiseptic solution or spray)

- Custom-made ice packs (unless ice is always readily available from a freezer or the freezing compartment of a refrigerator)

- Cotton wool, gauze swabs, surgical tape

- Scissors, tweezers and safety pins.

In addition the following are recommended for contact sports events and should be used only by someone trained to do so:

- Airways – small, medium and large

- Stretcher (scoop or foldable)

- Cervical collars – small, medium and large

- Inflatable and rigid splints.

[The Laerdal First Aid Kit is an excellent one.]

KEY POINTS

✓ Any bump on the head associated with memory loss or loss of consciousness should be regarded as serious and medical advice sought

✓ Learn basic life support techniques and principles because it could save someone's life

✓ Get medical help immediately whenever serious injury is suspected

Useful addresses

British Olympic Association
1 Wandsworth Plain
London SW18 1EH
Tel: 020 8871 2677
Fax: 020 8871 9104
Website: www.olympics.org.uk

National Olympic Committee which is responsible for all Olympic matters in the UK.

British Olympic Medical Institute
Northwick Park Hospital
Watford Road
Harrow
Middlesex HA1 3UJ
Tel: 020 8423 7200
Fax: 020 8423 7201

Provides medical facilities for Olympic athletes.

British Red Cross Society (England)
9 Grosvenor Crescent
London SW1X 7EJ
Tel: 020 7235 5454
Fax: 020 7245 6315
Email: information@redcross.org.uk
Website: www.redcross.org.uk

Gives skilled and impartial care to people in need and crisis in their own homes, the community, at home and abroad, in peace and in war. Refers to local branches.

British Red Cross Society (Scotland)
2 Swan Street
Glasgow G4 0AX
Tel: 0141 332 1607
Fax: 0141 332 5948
Email: information@redcross.org.uk
Website: www.redcross.org.uk

Gives skilled and impartial care to people in need and crisis in their own homes, the community, at home and abroad, in peace and in war. Refers to local branches.

Laerdal Medical Limited
Laerdal House
Goodmead Road
Orpington
Kent BR6 0HX
Tel: 01689 876634
Fax: 01689 873800
Email: customer.service@laerdal.co.uk
Website: www.laerdal.co.uk

Manufactures life-saving and training equipment, including mannequins.

National Sports Medicine Institute of the United Kingdom
32 Devonshire Street
London W1G 6PX
Tel: 020 7908 3636
Fax: 020 7908 3635
Email: enquiries@nsmi.org.uk
Website: www.nsmi.org.uk

Involved with other organisations and provides information, education and consultancy services for those engaged in exercise and sports.

Sport England
16 Upper Woburn Place
London WC1H 0QP
Tel: 020 7273 1500
Fax: 020 7273 1868
Email: info@english.sports.gov.uk
Website: www.sportengland.org

Government agency promoting sport in England with a wide variety of activity programmes in order to foster a healthier lifestyle.

Sport Scotland
Caledonia House
1 Redheughs Rigg
South Gyle
Edinburgh EH12 9DQ UK
Tel: 0131 317 7200
Fax: 0131 317 7202
Email: gen.info@sportscotland.org.uk
Website: www.sportscotland.org.uk

Government agency in Scotland promoting sport with a wide range of activity programmes.

Sportscoach UK
114 Cardigan Road
Headingley
Leeds LS6 3BJ
Tel: 0113 274 4802
Fax: 0113 275 5019
Email: coaching@sportscoachuk.org
Website: www.sportscoachuk.org

Develops coaches and coaching as a profession, working with a number of partners to improve sport throughout the UK.

Sports Council for Northern Ireland
House of Sport
Upper Malone Road
Belfast BT9 5LA
Tel: 02890 381222
Fax: 02890 682757
Email: info@sportni.net
Website: www.sportni.com

Government agency promoting sport in Northern Ireland with a wide variety of activity programmes.

Sports Council for Wales
Sophia Gardens
Cardiff CF1 9SW
Tel: 02920 300500
Fax: 02920 300600
Email: wis@scw.co.uk
Website: www.sports-council-wales.co.uk

Headquarters for national network of local clubs who arrange integrated projects to bring disabled and able-bodied people together. Promote sport in Wales and distribute lottery funding. Support Paralympic athletes.

St Andrew's Ambulance Association
St Andrew's House
Milton Street
Glasgow G4 0HR
Tel: 0141 332 4031
Fax: 0141 332 6582
Email: firstaid@staaa.demon.co.uk
Website: www.firstaid.org.uk

Provides first aid training and cover for events in Scotland.

St John's Ambulance
27 St John's Lane
London EC1M 4BU
Tel: 08702 355 231
Fax: 020 7324 4001
Helpline: 08700 104 950
Website: www.sja.org.uk

Provides first aid training and cover for events.

THE INTERNET AS A SOURCE OF FURTHER INFORMATION

After reading this book, you may feel that you would like further information on the subject. One source is the internet and there are a great many websites with useful information about medical disorders, related charities and support groups. Some websites, however, have unhelpful and inaccurate information. Many are sponsored by commercial organisations or raise revenue by advertising, but nevertheless aim to provide impartial and trustworthy health information. Others may be reputable but you should be aware that they may be biased in their recommendations. Remember that treatment advertised on international websites may not be available in the UK.

Unless you know the address of the specific website that you want to visit (for example familydoctor.co.uk), you may find the following guidelines helpful when searching the internet.

There are several different sorts of websites that you can use to look for information, the main ones being search engines, directories and portals.

Search engines and directories
There are many search engines and directories that all use different algorithms (procedures for computation) to return different results when you do a search. Search engines use computer programs called spiders, which crawl the web on a daily basis to search individual pages within a site and then queue them ready for listing in their database.

Directories, however, consider a site as a whole and use the description and information that was provided with the site when it was submitted to the directory to decide whether a site matches the searcher's needs. For both there is little or no selection in terms of quality of information, although engines and directories do try to impose rules about decency and content. Popular search engines in the UK include:

google.co.uk
aol.co.uk
msn.co.uk
lycos.co.uk
hotbot.co.uk
overture.com
ask.co.uk
espotting.com
looksmart.co.uk
alltheweb.com
uk.altavista.com

The two biggest directories are:

yahoo.com
dmoz.org

Portals

Portals are doorways to the internet that provide links to useful sites, news and other services, and may also provide search engine services (such as msn.co.uk). Many portals charge for putting their clients' sites high up in your list of search results. The quality of the websites listed depends on the selection criteria used in compiling the portal, although portals focused on a specific group, such as medical information portals, may have more rigorous inclusion criteria than other searchable websites. Examples of medical portals can be found at:

nhsdirect.nhs.uk
patient.co.uk

Links to many British medical charities will be found at the Association of Medical Research Charities (www.amrc.org.uk) and Charity Choice (www.charitychoice.co.uk).

Search phrases

Be specific when entering a search phrase. Searching for information on 'cancer' could give astrological information as well as medical: 'lung cancer' would be a better choice. Either use the engine's advanced search feature and ask for the exact phrase, or put the phrase in quotes – 'lung cancer' – as this will link the words. Adding 'uk' to your search phrase will bring up mainly British websites, so a good search would be 'lung cancer' uk (don't include uk within the quotes).

Always remember that the internet is international and unregulated. Although it holds a wealth of invaluable information, individual websites may be biased, out of date or just plain wrong. Family Doctor Publications accepts no responsibility for the content of links published in their series.

Index